Peace
FOR EACH
HOUR

BY MARY J. NELSON

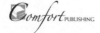

For information, address Comfort Publishing, 296 Church St. N., Concord, NC 28025. The views expressed in this book are not necessarily those of the publisher.

Unless otherwise indicated, all Scripture quotations are taken from the Holy Bible, New Living Translation, copyright ©1996, 2004, 2007 by Tyndale House Foundation. Used by permission of Tyndale House Publishers, Inc., Carol Stream, Illinois 60188. All rights reserved.

Scripture quotations marked (NIV) are taken from the Holy Bible, New International Version®, NIV®. Copyright © 1973, 1978, 1984, 2011 by Biblica, Inc.™ Used by permission of Zondervan. All rights reserved worldwide. www.zondervan.com The "NIV" and "New International Version" are trademarks registered in the United States Patent and Trademark Office by Biblica, Inc.™

Scripture taken from the New King James Version®. Copyright ©1982 by Thomas Nelson, Inc. Used by permission. All rights reserved.

Copyright ©2013 by Mary J. Nelson

First printing

Book cover design by Reed Karriker
Author photo by Dennis Chick

ISBN: 978-1-938388-17-0
Published by Comfort Publishing, LLC
www.comfortpublishing.com

Printed in the United States of America

Praise for *Peace for Each Hour*

"Peace for Each Hour by my friend Mary J. Nelson, might be the most encouraging book you'll ever read. God's promises, when proclaimed over our lives, will give us three powerful weapons to destroy and overcome fear: power, love, and a sound mind.

"What happens in you is more important than what happens to you! For all who need to strengthen themselves in the Lord, this book is for you."

Leif Hetland
President. Global Mission Awareness
Author of *Seeing Through Heaven's Eyes*

————

"But my journey took me to another place — a place of refreshing springs where pools of blessing collect after the rains" (p. 12). That's where Mary wants to take you. She writes with the voice of experience and the heart of compassion. She not only has a way with words, but she is intimately acquainted *with* the Word. So, again and again, her insights and wisdom offer encouragement and hope to survivors. Not just cancer survivors, but any who have come through the storms of life.

I.

"I love serving with Mary. She touches and teaches people in ways that make life better. This book will do the same for you."

Bill Bohline, Lead Pastor
Hosanna!

—◦◦◦—

"*Peace for Each Hour* is another masterpiece from Mary J. Nelson. Every page of it is filled with compassion, hope, and courage. In the Old Testament, God's glorious presence rested upon the Ark of Testimony before which Moses communed with God face to face. This furniture was made up of acacia wood overlaid with pure gold — a picture of humanity wrapped in divinity. Mary's journey of faith against cancer, her encounters with the Living Word through the process and her celebration of victory is a testament to this truth. To me, this book is an invitation for all to experience God's goodness and unfailing grace in the midst of pain, weaknesses, and discouragement. I highly recommend this book to all church leaders, counselors, and those who are going through 'the valley of the shadow of death'. The breath of God is on it. It tackles the topic of divine healing holistically, not as a theological discourse, but as an overflow of an honest straight-from-the-heart relationship with the Loving Father."

Paul Yadao, Lead Pastor
Destiny Ministries International

"I read Mary J. Nelson's most recent book *Peace for each Hour* while returning from a pastor's conference in India and was pleasantly surprised by the invaluable Kingdom principles that Mary has learned in her journey with Jesus through cancer. When I picked up the book, my first thought was I would have to get my mind "into" the cancer/suffering world on this long plane ride home. Wow, was I wrong! Mary has taken the timeless principles of how the Kingdom of God really works, all of which were learned through the cancer experience, and gotten "into" my world as she spoke in vignettes on various critical topics like faith, hope, grace, healing, doubt, fear, love, passion, etc. The book was loaded for me personally and as a pastor with useful strategies and mindsets that will help me coach others to win in whatever circumstances they may be challenged with. Not unlike the Christian classic *My Utmost for His Highest* by Oswald Chambers, it may also be one of the finest seminal books I have seen for preaching topics on the Kingdom of God! It was like an excellent buffet, the first time through it's about plate management, so you kind of sample. Now I'm headed back for the tasty and nutritional things I really want and need for me and others!"

Tim Hatt, Kingdom Expansion Pastor
Hosanna!

—◦◦◦—

"Mary J. Nelson has written another awesome book of encouragement to share with the multitudes of people whose lives are forever impacted by a cancer diagnosis. I have a twofold interest in this book. As Pastor of Care at a large church we encounter families daily in need of courage and hope. Personally I have survived ovarian, liver, and kidney cancer. We all search for and desire His peace rather than our fear. We hear of recurrences, surgeries, and treatments as well as live daily life alongside of others who do not win their personal earthly cancer battle. True peace is found in God's promises and the personal examples of others as shared in this book bringing emotional strength we all need to live a fruitful, happy, and peace-filled life. I look forward to not just enjoying this peace for myself but passing it on to many others in *Peace for Each Hour.*"

Pat Moe, Care Ministries Pastor
Hosanna!

———〰———

"Mary J. Nelson knows firsthand how hard it can be to overcome the oppression of illness and adversity. In her book *Peace for Each Hour* she shares with the reader brief words of encouragement that will help maintain focus on spiritual, emotional, and physical wholeness. I strongly recommend this book as an inspiration to anyone who needs to remember how big God really is."

Pastor Kristi Graner
Director, Dare To Believe Ministries
Regional Director, International Bethel Sozo

"A wonderful read from beginning to end. A journey with bumps in the road to the street of victory. I personally felt her struggles, her feelings. I could feel her hands clutching to the hem of His garment. Whatever your trial, this book will encourage you and cause you to keep your hand to the plow. A blessing to read *Peace for Each Hour.*"

Rev. Elaine C. Bonn, Director & President
Healing Center International
Minnesota Director, International Association of Healing Rooms

———❧———

"In *Peace for Each Hour,* Mary J. Nelson has written a devotional resource that is saturated with the literal word of God, pregnant and very richly anointed with the Holy Spirit. She allows the Word of God to speak for itself, while guiding the reader to the streams of living water and encouraging them to draw and drink that living word of healing, comfort, and faith. There are many Christian devotionals where the author and their ideas strive to become that living water to their readers. However, they fail to satisfy in this crucial process of recovery and healing. Mary has done the reverse. She brings the reader to the true source of healing and then fades into prayer, leaving the reader in the healing hands of Jesus through His word. The stories are touching, short and to the point, making the reader feel as if they are in someone's home around their kitchen table listening to their deep and sincere struggles, stories, and testimonies."

Dr. Gemechis Buba
Missions Director for the North American Lutheran Church and International Teacher, Preacher, and Leadership Consultant

"As a urologic surgeon, many of the patients I see daily are dealing with cancer. Although they typically put on a brave front, I can see the fear and anxiety in their eyes. As I counsel them on their illness, there is so much more I wish I could tell them. Mary J. Nelson has written an excellent devotional book that will help patients walk through their illness and beyond. Patients need to know that God is a loving Father and that He is bigger than their cancer. Through her book they will see that their identity is in Christ and not in the diagnosis they have been given. Putting their ultimate trust in the Great Physician will help them conquer their illness.

"The scientific literature has numerous studies documenting that cancer patients have better outcomes when they practice faith and prayer. *Peace for Each Hour* is an excellent book to help patients integrate their faith with their medical treatment. I recommend this book for anyone journeying through cancer."

Theodore J. Sawchuk MD, FACS
Urologic Surgeon, Fargo, ND

DEDICATION

This book is dedicated to Xavier and Lila
and all my future grandchildren; so thankful to know you
and love you on this side of Heaven.

May the peace of Christ guard your hearts and minds
from generation to generation.

ACKNOWLEDGEMENTS

Peace for Each Hour is my third published book. Like the others, it came from resting in a place of intimacy with God as He revealed more of His power, His presence, and His promises through my life experiences after cancer. There have many people who have shared these experiences with me. Some have spoken His truth into my life; some have taken the time to invest in me, while others have simply loved me for who I am, regardless of who I'm not. God is using all of them to mold and shape me so I can live in the fullness of Christ. For this, I'm profoundly grateful to:

My husband Howie; for 36 years you have loved me unconditionally through the highs and lows and the victories and defeats. I'm so blessed to grow in grace with you.

My children, son Bryan and daughter-in-law Sharmi, and daughter Kelly; I am grateful for the privilege of mothering you. You are all on a unique journey with God and I am so proud and thankful for who you have become and who God is preparing you to be.

Xsie and Lila; I always heard being a grandma was the best thing that could ever happen to me. I've learned it's better than that.

To my parents, Ray and Jeanne Hangge, my brother Mark and sister Marilyn; for your love, patience, and grace as God continues to transform me into the child He created. Remember, He has forgotten my past and He isn't finished with me yet!

My small group, Mary Carroll, Barb Wilson, and Julie Swecker; we've sharpened a lot of iron together and survived it all; I love you like sisters.

Chicks and the "up north gang;" for reminding me not to take this life too seriously and to find child-like delight in every blessing.

My ministry colleague, Pastor Mike Swecker; through all the challenges of ministry you have been my pastor, my Barnabas, and my steadfast friend. You have tested me with your adaptability while gently teaching me how to get out of the way and give God room to move.

Bill Bohline, Lead Pastor at Hosanna!; for your words "we believe the Lord led you here" and your church that changed my life forever.

Pat Moe, Care Pastor at Hosanna!; for teaching me how to pray and to comfort others with the same comfort God has given me.

Tim Hatt, Kingdom Impact Pastor at Hosanna!; for challenging me to step out of my comfort zone and to keep my eyes on the ultimate mission—advancing the Kingdom of God.

Pastor Kristi Graner; for inspiring me to step into my destiny as a pastor and for teaching me how to lead God's people to freedom.

Tony Caterina and the Pray for the Cure prayer team; for sharing your time and gifts with people battling cancer and for your unshakable faith in the healing promises of God.

To all the modern day forerunners and pioneers in the Kingdom whose books, ministries, and teachings have stirred my heart, including Leif Hetland, Paul Yadao, Randy Clark, Bill Johnson, Graham Cooke, Heidi Baker, Dutch Sheets, Cindy Jacobs, Mike Bickle, Joyce Meyer, and many, many more.

Finally, to Jason and Kristy Huddle, Reed Karriker, and the rest of the team at Comfort Publishing; for partnering with me in this book to help cancer survivors live victoriously, all for His glory.

TABLE OF CONTENTS

PREFACE

"I am leaving you with a gift—peace of mind and heart.
And the peace I give is a gift the world cannot give.
So don't be troubled or afraid. — John 14:27

Something life changing can happen when we brush against the door of death. A new normal replaces the old. The past can become an elusive memory and the future a place that can no longer be trusted. Just ask anyone who has survived military combat, a terrorist attack, a natural disaster, or a physical assault. Ask a cancer survivor. In the United States, there are over 11 million people living beyond the devastating diagnosis of cancer. Over two million of them survived breast cancer. People like Carla. As she struggles to prepare for life as a survivor, she vividly shares her deepest fear:

"I am a 34 year old mother of two diagnosed with stage 1 breast cancer. I have completed a bilateral mastectomy and four rounds of chemotherapy in December. I have been devastated! The fear of this cancer often takes over. My heart is heavy and confused, but I am trying to be strong and learn what faith and God are all about. I am struggling everyday and tired of being tired! The idea of having another PET or CT scan sends me to my knees. I don't know how people just sit and wait to see if cancer has taken over or has surprised them in some other spot.

I'm not even scheduled to be scanned until September, but I live every day in this waiting … waiting … waiting. I feel one step away from EVERYTHING truly being taken away."

If you're reading this book, you too may be a cancer survivor. Perhaps you've finished treatment and you're anxious to get on with your life, but you find yourself struggling with the same doubts and questions as Carla. *Will I ever be normal again? Will I always have this unsettled feeling that I'm only one step away from losing everything? After all, it happened once before and now I know I'm not immune. Will I ever be able to face those situations and places that bring back memories of my cancer treatment without shear panic taking my breath away? Will I always have this dark cloud of uncertainty hanging over me? Will this fear ever go away? Will I ever find peace again?*

The relief you experience when you walk away from a check up with a positive report can be exhilarating, but short-lived. You may have been blessed with the most brilliant minds and most advanced treatments in the medical realm to battle the cancer. But if you put your hope in the oncologists, their statistics, and the latest test results, the peace you crave will have you riding an emotional roller coaster of ups and downs. You'll find yourself living from check up to check up and test to test — filled with peace for a short while until the next appointment comes creeping up on your calendar.

There's a different kind of peace—a peace that surpasses all human understanding — a gift the world cannot give — a peace that never changes and never moves. It withstands the test of time. You can find this peace by traveling a higher road, one that soars above the clouds of uncertainty that threaten to darken your hopes and dreams. And this book will lead you there. Rich in the timeless truths of Scripture, 90 daily readings will reveal God's heart for you, His precious child. The Scripture references throughout the book will take you deeper into His Word for further understanding and revelation. Through His presence, His power, and His promises, He will lead you to a place of divine health where no test result and no doctor visit will move you, a place that knows no anxiety, no doubt, and no fear. May you have peace for each hour of the journey.

1

Now What?

I look up to the mountains – does my help come from there?
My help comes from the LORD, who made the heavens and the earth!
He will not let you stumble and fall; the one who watches over you
will not sleep. — Psalm 121:1-3

I walked out of the clinic clutching the "certificate of completion" the nurses had given it to me to celebrate the last day of a grueling journey through breast cancer treatment. It was a beautiful spring day and even nature was poised to join me in the celebration. Buds burst forth from the trees lining the boulevard and the sun shined brightly in the clear blue sky. I drew in a deep breath and everything smelled fresh and new. I should have been jumping and skipping and shouting praises to the heavens. But something was wrong. The routine that had become so familiar — the trips to the doctor who provided comfort and encouragement; the chemo drugs and radiation he used to kill the cancer; all the tests he ordered to monitor the results — everything that had consumed my life for the last eight months ended as abruptly as it started. All the weapons used to wage war against the enemy went back into the arsenal. My troops were in retreat. Suddenly, instead of doing something to fight back, I felt vulnerable and exposed.

Now what? Shortly after my diagnosis, I remember instinctively knowing that the most difficult time would come when the treatment ended. I knew my life would never be the same, and living as a survivor would require a new level of trust in the God who would carry me through the initial diagnosis and treatment. Now, I came face to face with that reality. From the depths of my soul, God whispered: "Where does your help truly come from? Where do you place your hope?" In the midst of the doctors and treatments and all the medical attention, our trust can slip so subtly from the Creator of the universe — the one and only Great Physician — to all the things He created. I became painfully aware that day of how much trust I had placed in the visible weapons of warfare when the outward battle abruptly ended.

What happens when the treatment ends, you are left feeling exposed and vulnerable, and the inner battle rages on? Will you look to the mountain and discover where your help really comes from? It comes from the Lord who created the heavens and the earth and brings the stars out one by one, calling each by name (Isaiah 40:26). It comes from the sovereign God who created your doctors, the miracle drugs, and all the medical breakthroughs. Everything good comes from Him and is intended for His glory (Romans 11:36; James 1:17). He keeps watch over you long after the weapons are put away and the troops retreat. He's been watching all along. He never tires and He never sleeps. Now what? Now it's just you and your God. If you can trust in the gifts that come directly from His hands, you can trust Him. The Lord Himself watches over you.

Father, thank you for watching over me through this journey. Help me to put my hope and trust in you the Creator, and not the weapons of this world. Amen.

2

His Word Stands

The grass withers, and the flowers fade beneath the breath of the LORD. And so it is with people. The grass withers, and the flowers fade, but the word of our God stands forever. — Isaiah 40:7-8

Diagnosis: Breast Cancer. Every year I would go in for my regular check up, these words appeared on the registration forms and orders I carried around the clinic. Year after year, the examination and tests showed no cancer. I would go in feeling healthy and well and very much alive. And every year, the same words appeared on my paperwork. Diagnosis: Breast Cancer. The words made me cringe. It's the same way I react when I hear someone say, "I'm in remission" or when I hear of a cancer support group led by someone "in remission." Remission is a term that is often misused. Remission implies I have cancer, but it's not actively growing and it might flare up at any minute without warning. I don't have cancer. I *had* cancer. Past tense.

For those who survive cancer, the voices of the world speak of recurrence rates and survival statistics. Not knowing which statistical group I might fall into, my doctors were cautious about proclaiming a "cure" when my treatment ended. Instead, they sent me home with resources on coping with an "uncertain future."

Their job is to look for signs of disease and they will continue to poke, prod, and stick me far into my so-called uncertain future, unconvinced of the physical evidence that continues to prove my health and wellness. I always feel a little bit like I'm on trial in a backward justice system, where instead of "innocent until proven guilty," I'm "sick until proven well."

In contrast, the Word of God speaks life, healing, and hope into the world. In Him, my future is certain, filled with good and not disaster (Jeremiah 29:11). The enemy seeks to steal, kill, and destroy life, but He has come to give me life in all its fullness (John 10:10). Even in the midst of affliction and sorrow, He has overcome the world and all its trials (John 16:33). He personally carried my sins and sickness in His own body on the cross. By His stripes I am healed (1 Peter 2:24)! When Thomas demanded physical proof that He had conquered death, our Lord simply reached our His nail-scarred hands and said, "You believe because you have seen me. Blessed are those who haven't seen me and believe anyway" (John 20:24-30). In living my life after cancer, I choose certainty, not doubt. I choose hope, not despair. I choose Jesus. I choose to listen to His voice over the other voices of the world.

When the world treats you like you still have cancer and your future is uncertain, will you agree? Will you live the rest of your life under dark clouds of doubt, never certain you are really healed, just waiting for the enemy to rise up and confirm your worst fear? Or will you come into agreement with the Word of God? God's Word promises to give you back your health and heal your wounds (Jeremiah 30:17). By His tender mercies, He forgives all your sins and heals all your diseases (Psalm 103:2-3). The grass withers and the flowers fade, and the medical realm and all its wonders will pass away. In spite of what the world may tell you, today, tomorrow, or at next year's check up, His Word stands forever.

Father, thank you for your Word that speaks life and stands the test of time. Help me to listen and agree with your voice over all the other voices of the world. Amen.

3

WAITING FOR THE OTHER SHOE

*Who else has held the oceans in his hand? Who has measured off
the heavens with his fingers? Who else knows the weight of the
earth or has weighed out the mountains and the hills?
Who is able to advise the Spirit of the LORD? Who knows enough to
be his teacher or counselor?* — Isaiah 40:12-13

"At least you know how you're going to die." Excuse me? I
couldn't believe my ears. She was only trying to console me after
a recent breast cancer diagnosis. But her comment struck a nerve
and continues to creep back into my mind occasionally as I live my
life as a survivor. On the other side of cancer, every ache and pain
takes on new meaning when we presume to fully know the mind of
God. If I discount His sovereign power and His saving grace — if
I never truly believe in His unfailing love for me — naturally I'll
sit around waiting for the other shoe to drop. I can easily allow
cancer to become my identity and the nemesis that defines me.
I can continue let it consume my thoughts and steal my hopes
and dreams, because now I know the plan. My ticket is already
punched.

No, my God is bigger than cancer and I won't let it define me.
My identity comes from my Father who created me and watched as

I was woven together in the darkness of the womb (Psalm 139:14-15). It comes from His Son who suffered a cruel death for my mistakes and the sins of the world (Romans 3:24-25). And it comes from the Holy Spirit who lives in me and gives me comfort (John 14:16-18). I know that only by His gracious favor I live, and move, and exist (Acts 17:28). I am His masterpiece and He created me with a purpose (Ephesians 2:10). Each day of my life was written in His book, each moment planned out before a single day had passed (Psalm 139:16). His plans for my life are more wonderful than anything my limited human mind can imagine (Isaiah 55:8-9). My God held the oceans in His hands. How can I possibly understand His decisions, His methods, or what He is thinking (Romans 11:33-34)? Yet, by seeking His presence and spending time in His Word, I can begin to know His character. I can gain insight into His will for my future (John 16:13-15). I can talk to Him through prayer and expect Him to answer (1 Corinthians 2:16). I can come to know Him personally and experience His unfailing love for me (John 14:21).

Are you waiting for the other shoe to drop? When you let cancer define your identity, a headache isn't just a headache — it's brain metastases. Every backache sends you into a panic. A dark cloud of doubt footnotes every hope and every dream. But if you call Jesus your Lord and Savior, you belong to Him, not to the whim of cancer (Ephesians 2:13). You can trust Him to govern your life with wisdom, justice, and love. Through Him, you can find peace in any circumstance (John 14:27). Through Him, you can have overflowing joy (John 15:11). Through Him, you can have life in all its fullness (John 10:10). No, you may not always know what tomorrow will bring. But I guarantee, you will find a better life in Jesus than you will ever find waiting for the other shoe.

Father, thank you that my identity is only in you. Help me to grasp the scope of your awesome power and love and to trust in you alone. Amen.

4

THE NEW "WHY ME?"

"My thoughts are completely different from yours," says the LORD.
"And my ways are far beyond anything you could imagine.
For just as the heavens are higher than the earth, so are my ways
higher than your ways and my thoughts higher than your thoughts."
— Isaiah 55:8-9

I used to wonder why. Why did I get breast cancer? I have healthy parents and grandparents who lived well into the eighties and nineties. I had no relevant family history. Sometimes I'm convinced it was my stressful work schedule, my perfectionist personality, my poor eating habits, and the fact that I never drank water. Now that I'm several years on the other side, there's a new spin on the same old question. Why did I survive and my friend didn't? Why am I healthy while another person battles advanced disease? Everyone is quick to offer an opinion on the subject. It must be your positive attitude. You must have had stronger chemo and a better doctor. You must be taking the right vitamin supplements. You have a wonderful family and good Christian friends to love and support you. It must be your strong faith!

It's our human nature to wonder why. The disciples thought they knew the answer — sin. "Teacher, why was this man born blind? Was it a result of his own sins or those of his parents?" they asked. Jesus simply answered, "He was born blind so the power of God could be seen in him" (John 9:2-3). And He promptly healed him. Peter wondered about God's sense of fairness. When Jesus revealed the kind of death he would eventually suffer to glorify God, Peter wanted to know what God's plans were for John, the other disciple. "What about him, Lord?" Jesus told Peter it was none of his business. Peter's only responsibility was to seek and know Jesus. "If I want him to remain alive until I return, what is that to you? You follow me "(John 21:18-23).

We want to understand God's physical creation and how things work. We want to understand His mind perfectly. In reality, we understand neither. Job came to that stark realization when God challenged him with a series of questions as he sat broken and covered with boils, everything of value stripped away. "Where were you when I laid the foundations of the earth? Tell me if you know so much," His voice boomed from the heavens (Job 38:4). We all tend to pull God down to our own limited understanding of justice and fairness. We compare our lives with others, either to rationalize our own righteousness or to question God's sense of justice. But His ways and His thoughts are higher than ours. Job was a righteous man before he suffered and God restored his life. Yet Job came to understand it was far better to know God than to know why. When we start making our need to know why a condition of our faith in Him — when we want to understand His ways more than we desire Him — we miss out on everything else God wants to reveal to us through a personal relationship with His Son.

Never let your inability to understand His ways cause you to doubt the promises of God or hinder your relationship with Him.

His love for you is limitless and His plans for you are perfect. You can trust Him to fit all the puzzle pieces of life into a complete and perfect picture and reveal it in His appointed time and way. In the meantime, in the midst of all the things you wonder, there is one thing you can count on — God is using your journey for His good purposes (Romans 8:28). Perhaps cancer brought you to a personal saving faith in Jesus Christ. Perhaps through your healing, others see His glory. Perhaps you'll never know. But you don't need to know why. The answers lie far beyond anything you could imagine, as far as the heavens rise above the earth. You don't need to fully understand His ways. You only need to know Him.

Father, thank you that your ways and thoughts are higher than mine. Forgive me if I've made understanding you a condition of my faith. Help me to give up the need to know. Amen.

5

One Way Ticket

...for he called you out of the darkness into his wonderful light.
"Once you were not a people; now you are the people of God.
Once you received none of God's mercy; now you have received his
mercy." Dear brothers and sisters, you are foreigners and aliens here.
— 1 Peter 2:9-11

I finally reached the end of a long unplanned journey through the wilderness. My itinerary had taken me through waiting rooms, hospital laboratories, operating rooms, chemo clinics, and wig shops. My tour guides tried to make me as comfortable as possible as they poked, prodded, stuck, infused, and radiated me at every turn. But my journey took me to another place — a place of refreshing springs where pools of blessing collect after the rains (Psalm 84:6)! It was in this place I received supernatural comfort in the most hopeless of days. It was here in my brokenness where He revealed His remarkable secrets (Jeremiah 33:3). It was here where God called me out of the darkness and into His wonderful light and poured out His mercy. In this place, Jesus Christ won my heart.

By His grace, I reached the end of the long and arduous journey. As I stood at the edge of the wilderness looking back at the path

I had walked, I was struck by the realization that I made the trip alone. My family and friends, those who loved me and supported me, didn't make the same trip. Yes, we shared in the itinerary. They traveled alongside me through all the difficult decisions, treatments, and clever head coverings. But they didn't come with me to that place in the wilderness — that place of refreshing springs — where Jesus met my unspoken needs. To many who know and love me, my journey is over. But they never stood with me at the end of my humanness where my own strength was no longer enough. They didn't meet death face to face. They never lived with me week after week, month after month, in that dark bald place, with every hope and dream stripped away — clinging only to Jesus. He was my hope, my source of comfort, and the only one who really understood. By His grace, I continue my journey through life after cancer, trusting everyday to His care and protection. My love and devotion for Jesus seems impassioned and desperate because He has faithfully met my most desperate needs (Luke 7:47).

As a survivor, you may feel like a stranger in a world that doesn't understand what you've been rescued from. You may feel surrounded by people who don't know or understand the one who rescued us all. This should come as no surprise. As Christ followers, we are foreigners and aliens in this world. Our real citizenship is in Heaven (Philippians 3:20). His Kingdom came to earth in the life of Jesus Christ and spread to every believer through the gift of the Holy Spirit. Once He lifted you out of the pit of destruction and set your feet on solid ground, there's no turning back (Psalm 40:2). God has chosen you as His very own child. He has shown you His mercy. You can go directly into His throne room with every thought and every need (Hebrews 4:16). He is the only one who truly understands. Sure, you may be mocked, misunderstood, or criticized by those who don't. You may even feel like an alien here. Take heart. You have a one-way ticket to the Kingdom of God.

Father, thank you calling me out of the darkness and into your Kingdom of Light. Help me to trust everyday in this foreign land to your care and protection. Amen.

6

His Sovereign Hand

The LORD has said to me in the strongest terms: "Do not think like everyone else does. Do not be afraid that some plan conceived behind closed doors will be the end of you. Do not fear anything except the LORD Almighty. He alone is the Holy One. If you fear him, you need fear nothing else. He will keep you safe. — Isaiah 8:11-14

Every year, it was the same clinic, the same routine exam, the same mammogram, and the same result. Negative. But this year, as the time came to schedule the annual visit, a silent voice at the core of my soul began to nudge me. It's time for a change. I had no idea why, but I listened. I reached out to the best minds in my "every woman's network" and they unanimously recommended a wonderful woman doctor considered to be one of the best in her field. She was so wonderful, she was booked a year in advance. It didn't matter. She wasn't taking new patients. I reluctantly scheduled an appointment with one of her colleagues. It was still several months out, so I asked to be added to the cancellation wait list.

I didn't wait long. The very next day the receptionist called. There was an opening, but not with Dr. Wonderful's colleague. It was with Dr. Wonderful herself. There was a scheduling miscue and she had failed to book the doctor's entire day. Could I come in tomorrow? Yes, she knew I was a new patient, but it was short notice and they would make an exception. I knew at that very moment — this year would not be the same. The mammogram was still negative. But this Dr. Wonderful found something slightly suspicious. She ordered more tests and the rest is history. I became the poster child for "breast cancer doesn't always present itself in the way we expect."

Throughout the next year and my life after cancer, I've taken great comfort in knowing God's hand was in this journey from the very beginning. It would have been easy to miss His presence in all the commotion. It would have been easy to assume He didn't care. But He spoke to me in the strongest terms through my circumstances. This plan the enemy conceived behind closed doors would not be the end of me. He promised to keep me safe. His sovereign hand delivered me just in time to the doctor who would find the cancer. The God who made me would certainly not bail on me in the weeks, months, and years to come (1 Peter 4:19). He promised He would never leave me or forsake me (Hebrews 13:5).

If you ask Him, God will show you His sovereign hand in every detail of your journey. After all, this storm didn't catch your Creator by surprise. He watched you being formed in the darkness of the womb. He laid out every moment of your life before a single day had passed. He walked before you when this cancer struck and beside you during your treatment. He both precedes and follows you as you walk into your future (Psalm 139:5, 15-16). Look for Him in the details that led to your diagnosis. See His sovereign hand in the wonderful doctor who cares for you, the timing of the new drugs He created, the people who love and encourage you, and all the ways He continues to use this cancer for His good purposes. Keep listening to the Lord when He speaks through your circumstances. His sovereign hand will keep you safe.

Father, thank you that your sovereign hand is in every detail of my life. Help me to see your comforting presence in all my circumstances. Amen.

7

SET FREE

And you will know the truth, and the truth will set you free.
— John 8:32

It was the strangest thing. It was a supernatural presence I couldn't explain. I felt it next to me in the car on the way to the very first appointment, and from that moment on, I couldn't escape it. It sat with me while I waited for examinations, biopsies, ultrasounds, and x-rays. It stood guard as my arm was stuck repeatedly and infused with powerful drugs. It followed me into laboratories and examination rooms where I was poked, palpated, and left to wait for test results. It watched by my bedside during the night and greeted me every morning. This invisible presence shadowed me around the house as if it had marching orders. In all my comings and goings, it never left my side. Eventually, the journey ended and life slowly returned to a semblance of normal. Suddenly one day, I noticed it was gone.

All through the cancer journey, I found comfort in the Psalms. One of my favorites promised if I made the Lord my refuge and the Most High my shelter, no evil will conquer me, and no plague will come near my dwelling. He will order his angels to protect me wherever I go and they will hold me safe in their hands (Psalm

91:9-12). I sensed that comfort and protection by my side at every turn. I had grown accustomed to it. It was like another person in the room, but one I couldn't see. Sometimes, I thought I was dreaming. But now, it was gone and I knew it was real. I asked God to help me understand.

The answer came at worship one night. The teaching was on Peter's arrest during the Passover celebration. King Herod imprisoned him, bound him in chains, and planned to put him on trial and execute him. The believers prayed earnestly for Peter's safety and God answered. Suddenly, there was a bright light in the cell. An angel of the Lord woke Peter and the chains fell off his wrists. The angel told him to get dressed follow him. Peter obeyed, but all the time he thought he was dreaming. He followed the angel past the guard posts, through the prison gate, and out into the street. *And then the angel suddenly left him* (Acts 12:7).

Just as reality struck Peter, the meaning of these words penetrated the core of my soul. The angel left Peter because he was free! Free from harm, free from judgment, and free from death at the hands of Herod. And I was free from the chains of cancer. But there was more. The cancer that held me in solitary confinement was the very thing that brought me to the foot of the cross. Before Jesus, I was a prisoner to my sin with no hope of escape. But now, I'm free from judgment and death because Jesus shed His blood and died for me. My faith in Him made me right with God, free from the consequences of sin and the lies of the enemy. God's angelic messenger stood guard in my prison, but His hand guided and protected me through my journey to know the truth. And the angel left me because now I'm free — free to follow God and be all that He meant for me to be.

Has the angel left you? It doesn't matter who you are or what you have done. In His mercy, He orchestrated the perfect escape plan. He sent His Son to rescue you. It is only by God's grace and infinite love that you are saved. Receive His free gift of life (Romans 3:20-25; Ephesians 2:8-10; John 3:16). Follow Him through the prison gate and discover all you were created to be. No, you're not dreaming. The chains are gone. His truth has set you free.

Father, thank you for guiding and protecting me and never leaving my side. My chains are gone and I am free! Help me to follow you into a future of hope and purpose. Amen.

8

Mind Games

The weapons we fight with are not the weapons of the world.
On the contrary, they have divine power to demolish strongholds.
We demolish arguments and every pretension that sets itself up against
the knowledge of God, and we take captive every thought to make it
obedient to Christ. — 2 Corinthians 10:4-5 (NIV)

During treatment, the battle for survival was fought in the doctor's office, the operating room, and the chemo clinic. Now, the battle is fought in my mind. As time passes, there are fewer mental skirmishes. But even several years later, the enemy tries to tempt me with his little mind games. It happened every year as I retraced familiar steps through the clinic parking ramp and up the elevator to the oncologist's office. It escalated into full scale battle while I waited forever for her to come into the examining room. It can still happen sometimes when I'm day dreaming about watching my grandchildren grow up and the fun things we can do together as a family. Occasionally, it can happen when I'm praying for someone who needs a miracle. *Do you really think this is all behind you? Do you really believe your God can heal?*

Whether or not I play these games depends on who I allow to control my mind. God has given me weapons to demolish every lie that would keep my thoughts from aligning with His. He gave me the Holy Spirit and when I choose daily to let Him control my mind, there is always life and peace (Romans 8:6). God's peace is completely different than the world's peace. The relief that comes from this year's check up is a temporary peace. It only lasts until the time for next year's check up draws near. God's peace is eternal and forever. It comes from knowing He controls my destiny — not yesterday's cancer, today's headache, or tomorrow's test results. When the enemy tries to play his little mind games and steal my peace, my best weapon against him is prayer. God promises a peace far more wonderful than my human mind can understand when I turn all my worries into prayers of petition and thanks. Reading Scripture every day helps keep my thoughts submitted to His authority and focused on what is right and true. There is no fear I can encounter in this life, either before or after cancer that God doesn't tackle in His Word. There is no lie His Son hasn't defeated. If I believe He is Lord and put His weapons and promises into practice, the peace of God will be assured (Philippians 4:6-9).

If the enemy is playing mind games with you, it's time to take back control. You have all the power of God behind you. You have prayer when worries come. You have the Word of God at your disposal. And you have faith and hope in Jesus Christ. Since you have been raised to new life with Him, you are free to set your sights on the realities of Heaven. You thoughts are not bound to the things here on earth (Colossians 3:1-2). There's no point in engaging in little mind games with the enemy. Your God is Commander over the battle in your mind. He has already won every game the enemy would entice you to play. Submit every thought that would disrupt your peace into His divine control. Let the enemy know you're through playing games.

Father, thank you for the weapons you have given me to demolish every lie that would keep my thoughts from aligning with yours. Help to hold every thought captive to your authority alone. Amen.

9

Hold Your Ground

"From eternity to eternity I am God. No one can oppose what I do. No one can reverse my actions." — Isaiah 43:13

I had the best treatment available for Stage 2 breast cancer. It was the "gold standard" of its time for the cancer cells described on my pathology report — the ideal combination of chemotherapy drugs, administered in just the right amounts and just the right intervals. It wasn't long before the media and the journal services began reporting new regimens and different agents for the same type of cancer. At first, I felt a twinge of panic. Oh no, I didn't get that treatment! Eventually, I came to terms with the fast paced reality of medical science. Forty years ago, doctors didn't even use chemo. They performed radical mastectomies and crossed their fingers. Forty years from now, breast cancer could be like polio or smallpox. Prevention could be as simple as a childhood immunization.

Yes, our brilliant human doctors and their medical breakthroughs have much to offer when we're sick and desperate. If I give all the credit to the doctors who treated me and the treatments they used — if I put all my hopes for a healthy future into their hands — I'm in big trouble. Their standards and methods change along with a changing world. But there is one who never changes (Malachi

3:6). He is the Alpha and the Omega — the Ruler of the past, present, and future — and the Beginning and the End of all existence (Revelations 1:8). He is the same yesterday, today, and forever (Hebrews 13:8). I don't want to place my trust in a healing that came from minds and methods that are here today and gone tomorrow. I want to trust a healing that came directly from the hands of a God who never changes. Because whatever God does is final. Nothing can be added to it or taken from it (Ecclesiastes 4:13). No one can oppose what He does or reverse His actions. The enemy might try to convince me otherwise, but he cannot take back a healing that came directly from the hand of God.

Who do you thank and praise for your healing? Perhaps you had brilliant doctors who used the most cutting edge cancer treatments available. You may feel deeply indebted to them for saving your life. But in just a few short years, there will be a new gold standard and those same treatments will be out of date. Your God is never out of date and He doesn't change His mind. When the news stories report the latest breakthroughs, don't panic. Remember who controls the medical realm and all its wonder. Remember who ultimately orchestrated your healing and give your thanks to Him alone. No one can reverse His actions. If the enemy threatens to take back what your God has won for His glory, hold your ground.

Father, thank you that you are the same yesterday, today, and forever. Help me to keep my trust focused on you, my Healer, and not the world around me. Amen.

10

Do You Love Him?

Once more he asked him, "Simon son of John, do you love me?"
Peter was grieved that Jesus asked the question a third time. He said,
"Lord, you know everything. You know I love you." — John 21:17

I'm a mom. Even though my kids have left the nest and have homes and children of their own, they still need me. They wonder who to call to prepare their income taxes, apply for a mortgage, or fix the furnace. They need my help with their kids, my recipes, my tips for handling insurance and car repairs after a fender bender, and my help deciding what to buy Dad for Christmas. I like to be needed. But I long for something more. I long for my children to want to hang out with me and simply enjoy my company — not because I'm Mom and they need something from me — just because they love me for the person I am.

When Jesus was arrested, Peter denied knowing Him three times, exactly as the Lord said he would do. After His resurrection, Jesus pressed Peter again. Three times, He asked, "Do you love me?" The first two times He used the Greek word "agape" describing a self-sacrificial divine love offered by choice. But the third time, He used the Greek word "phileo," a brotherly love with shared affection. In effect, Jesus was asking Peter if he was even His friend. Jesus put His finger on the heart of the matter and Peter was grieved. "Lord, you know all things." Jesus forced Peter to confront his true feelings about Him, and it saddened Peter that he didn't yet love Him with an agape love.

Do we really love Jesus for who He is or do we love Him for what we need from Him? My husband tells a wonderful story when he ministers to the unemployed. He starts by drawing a large capital "J" for "Job" on the board as he shares his 14-month journey through unemployment. He describes all the strategies and techniques he used to land the perfect job. He was a finalist many times, but as each job opportunity fell through his fingers, he fell further and further into a pit of despair. He eventually found his job, but not before He discovered he needed another "J" word even more. He needed Jesus. The Lord became more than his Provider. He became his beloved Friend. When breast cancer dropped me into the same dark pit, the Lord reached down and pulled me out. I needed healing and He came to my rescue. But I needed Jesus more. As I continue to seek Him with all my heart and soul, I know Him as Friend. I long for the times when I can just hang out with Him, enjoy His presence, and expect nothing in return. And I know He is pleased with my total devotion and my undivided attention. I know He wants me to love Him more than life itself (Luke 14:26).

Jesus challenged the nature of Peter's love and He challenges us. When Jesus was crucified, He didn't entrust the care of His mother to his brothers. He entrusted her care to John, the one disciple who risked staying with Him at the cross when all the others scattered (John 19:26). Can you love the Lord your God that much? Do want to reach a place where you want Jesus more than your health? More than life itself? As His follower, you are His disciple. Jesus regards all His disciples as friends. Just imagine having the King of Kings as your own personal friend. He's so eager to make everything known to you (John 15:15). He offers intimate friendship with those who revere Him, and with them, He shares His most treasured secrets (Psalm 25:14). Spend some time in His presence today. He longs for your love and devotion. Simply enjoy His company — not because He's God and you need something from Him — but just because you love Him.

Father, thank you that your Son is both my Savior and Friend. Lord, help me to want you more than anything I need from you. Help me to love with agape love. Amen.

11

THE DOCTOR IS ALWAYS IN

And I am sure that God, who began the good work within you, will continue his work until it is finally finished on that day when Christ Jesus comes back again. — Philippians 1:6

When the Great Physician walked on this earth, the crowds clamored around Him hoping for a touch or a word from Him that would restore their crippled legs, give them back their sight, and heal their diseases (Matthew 14:34-35). Many came to believe He was the Messiah as they received and witnessed His healing miracles. Even today, the world flocks to Doctor Jesus when difficulties are too great to be surmounted any other way. A health crisis like cancer often brings us to the very end of ourselves and becomes the impetus for the seeds of our faith to take root. If we fall to our knees in desperation seeking a Savior, we will always find Him (Matthew 7:8). After a healing touch from Doctor Jesus, will you stay there? As the months and years pass, will you stay on your knees and continue to seek Him with all your heart and soul?

As time passes and a healthy lifestyle gradually replaces the time consumed by cancer treatments and doctoring, we can easily slip back to our old ways. Perhaps, like the nine lepers, we received our healing and never gave another thought to coming back (Luke

17:12-17). Maybe we believe Jesus is more like a highly specialized physician who is only interested in hearing from us when we're facing a life threatening crisis. Even when our cancer journey left us with a deep longing to know Him better, our busy schedules can quickly crowd out our daily quiet times with the Lord. We may not read the Bible as often, or find time to spend with Him in prayer every day. When faced with competing priorities, we can let our fellowship with Jesus slip. Without even realizing it, we've quietly fallen outside the Lord's protection. We no longer rest in His shadow where He is our refuge and our shield (Psalm 91:1-4).

Jesus promised protection, but we must be abiding in the Spirit to experience it fully. If we stay connected to Him as a branch connects to a vine — if His words remain in us — our prayers will be heard and answered (John 15:5-7). When we abide in His presence through our daily fellowship and devotion, our hearts are perfectly in tune with His. And He shields and protects those who are faithful and loyal to Him (Psalm 31:23; Proverbs 2:7). Think of it as a God-sized "extended warranty" on the work He began when we first believed.

The moment you invited Jesus into the cancer, He began to mold you into the masterpiece He created. He began preparing you to do the good things He planned for you long ago (Ephesians 2:8-10). He never intended for you to receive your healing and walk away until the next insurmountable problem comes along. In fact, He cautions you not to drift away from the assurance you received when you first heard the Good News and to stand in it firmly (Colossians 1:23). He wants to guide and protect you and finish what He started. You don't need a special appointment or a life threatening crisis to see Him. The Doctor is always in.

Father, thank you for sending Doctor Jesus to rescue me when my troubles seem insurmountable. Help me to live daily in your presence and stand firmly in my faith so you can finish the good work you began. Amen.

12

BABY STEPS

The steps of the godly are directed by the LORD. He delights in every detail of their lives. Though they stumble, they will not fall, for the LORD holds them by the hand. — Psalm 37:23-24

I had a tendency to get way ahead of God. My "life plan" included everything from how many children I would like to have, their ideal genders, and of course, their names. I carefully planned out every career move, where we would live, what our house would look like, and what we would do for family fun. I mapped out our finances so we could educate our kids in private colleges, pay off the mortgage, and retire with plenty of time and money left to do the things we enjoy. Cancer was a big black unexpected thunder cloud that dumped buckets of rain on my hopes and dreams. I emerged from the storm into the calm warm sunlight with a very different life plan.

It took some time before I could speak out loud the words "I'm a cancer survivor" or say, "next year we should go…" without an eerie sense of foreboding. It felt like I was speaking without official authorization. Our natural tendency is to plan, hope, and dream. God made us that way. But He wants to be at the center of our planning. He wants to direct our steps (Proverbs 16:9). Before cancer came and darkened the sky, I had a bad habit of leaving Him out. Even when I knew my goals were God-ordained, I could grow impatient and take matters in my own hands. Now I'm learning His timing is perfect. The Israelites wandered the desert for forty years, but they learned not to budge until the cloud that hovered above them began to move. It was their signal to pack up camp and follow. God was on the move. Now I know that even when the cloud overhead turns dark and unexpected storms come, God can use these times to teach me obedience, build my faith, and reveal His character as I lean on Him.

Today, as you stand under the clear blue sky, you are grateful the storm has passed. But you want more. You want to be certain the storm clouds will never return to darken another day. You want answers. You want Him to light up the sky and let you see into your future. You want to know where you're going and how you'll get there. But God won't reveal all the answers. He'll give you something much better. He'll reveal Himself to you. As you spend time with your heavenly Daddy and share your hopes and dreams with Him, you'll discover He has wonderful plans for your life (Jeremiah 29:11). But He wants you to trust your plans to Him. Because His plans are bigger and better than anything you could ever dream or imagine (Isaiah 55:8-9). And like the best of parents, He will do things His way. Step by step, He directs your way. Step by step, He delights in every detail. Even when you stumble, He won't let you fall. No long strides. No running ahead of the cloud. One small step at a time. Baby steps.

Father, thank you that your plans are perfect and you never let me fall. Help me to leave the timing and the details up to you because you delight in me! Amen.

13

A Happy Song

For the LORD your God has arrived to live among you.
He is a mighty savior. He will rejoice over you with great gladness.
With his love, he will calm all your fears. He will exult over you
by singing a happy song." — Zephaniah 3:17

It's over. No more needle sticks and bruised arms. No more waiting in the big chair for hours watching people, watching the clock, and watching the bag of powerful chemicals hanging on the IV stand as it slowly empties into your body. No more blood tests and shots to boost your white count. No more two hour daily jaunts to the clinic to receive two minutes of radiation. No more hats, wigs, scarves, and eyebrow pencils. Maybe now, you can put your life back together. Maybe now, you can be happy again. And you are — until the first check up, the first scan, the first blood draw — and the next one and the next. You may wonder if this cancer, even though it's behind you, will always try to steal your joy. Will there always be that underlying caution deep inside? Will you never again let your guard down and allow yourself to get too comfortable?

As we journey through life, we eventually discover that true happiness isn't dependent on our circumstances or the events we can't control. On the contrary, achieving joy through a perfect problem free life is an elusive goal. No, true happiness comes from a consistent personal relationship with the Risen Lord. In fact, Jesus said if we stay connected with Him in thought, through His Word, and in prayer — if we simply remain in His presence and bask in His love — our joy will overflow (John 15:7-11)!

The Apostle Paul understood this kind of joy. He learned to be happy in every situation, whether extreme poverty, abundant wealth, physical pain or imprisonment (Philippians 4:11-13). Jesus filled all the empty places in Paul's life — his deepest longings — to full and overflowing. Paul was grateful for everything God had given Him. His contentment came from his relationship with Jesus, his only source of power. The happiness that comes through living daily with Jesus cannot be shaken — not by devastating lows or deceptive highs — not by blood tests, bone scans, mammograms or by any other circumstance.

Perhaps in that dark place of your past, you discovered your true Source of happiness. When you invited Him into the middle of the cancer, the Lord your God arrived to live with you forever. True joy comes when the Holy Spirit dwells in you and controls your life (Galatians 5:20). Follow Him and obey His commands. Know Him, love Him, and remember Him always. He is your Mighty Savior. Regardless of your circumstances, He will rejoice over you with great gladness. He will calm all your fears with His unfailing love. The God of all creation dances over you today. Can you hear? He's singing a happy song!

Father, thank you calming my fears with your love and rejoicing over me with singing. Help me to know you as the true Source of happiness and joy, regardless of my circumstances. Amen.

14

HIS UNSHAKABLE KINGDOM

This means that the things on earth will be shaken, so that only eternal things will be left. Since we are receiving a Kingdom that cannot be destroyed, let us be thankful and please God by worshiping him with holy fear and awe. For our God is a consuming fire.
— Hebrews 12:27-29

I never gave much thought to my mortality. I was still relatively young, healthy, and living on what I thought was the top of the world when cancer gave me a wakeup call. I was barely on the other side of the journey when airplanes slammed into tall buildings killing thousands of innocent Americans and setting off an international campaign to stop terrorists from destroying our peace and freedom. Even if these efforts prove successful, no amount of military might can stop a tsunami from killing nearly 300,000 people in Southeast Asia, an earthquake from killing nearly a half million people in Pakistan, Haiti, and Japan, or the hurricanes that crash relentlessly into the Florida and Gulf coasts destroying everything in their path, including an entire U.S. city. Add oil spills, poverty, record unemployment, an economic downturn and a crumbling world economy into the mix and we are easily living in the most unsettling of times.

Even in the worst catastrophe imaginable, believers have no cause for concern. We stand on a solid foundation that can never be destroyed. Jesus is the secret to weathering any storm, whether yesterday's cancer or the uncertain future that lies ahead. Anyone who listens and obeys His teaching is wise like a person who builds a house on solid rock. Though the rain comes in torrents and the floodwaters rise and the winds beat against it, the house won't collapse. But anyone who hears and ignores His teaching is like a person who builds a house on sand. When the rains and floods come and the winds beat against it, the house falls with a mighty crash (Matthew 7:24-27). Someday, the entire world will be shaken and only the eternal things of God will be left standing. But even then, we have nothing to fear. We belong to a Kingdom that can never be shaken, no matter what the future brings.

Are you building your house on rock or sand? Do you put your hope in the powers of this world, or an eternal Kingdom that can never be destroyed? The world seeks ways to stop the tide. But like a raging fire, God is not in your control. He cannot be contained or forced to do your bidding. Yet, He is good, a God of deep compassion whose love for you is limitless. His Son died to make you a citizen of Heaven. His sacrifice saved you from sin and will save you from death. Only what is dedicated to Him will endure the sifting and the shaking. Only what stands on Christ's firm foundation will last. On that glorious day, His Kingdom will come out of Heaven like a beautiful bride prepared for her husband. God himself will live among you in a place where there is no more death or sorrow or crying or pain. The old world and its evils will be gone forever (Revelation 21:2-4). Listen and obey His teaching. Worship Him today with holy fear and awe. Stand firm on the Rock. In His unshakable Kingdom, your life endures forever.

Father, thank you for your Kingdom that cannot be destroyed, regardless of what the future might bring. I stand on the Rock! Help me to focus my hope only on eternal things. Amen.

15

SEND ME

Then I heard the LORD asking, "Whom should I send as a messenger to my people? Who will go for us?" And I said, "LORD, I'll go! Send me." — Isaiah 6:8

Isaiah had a respectable career as a scribe in the royal palace in Jerusalem before God revealed His plans. Through a life changing vision where he encountered God personally, God called Isaiah and commissioned Him to be a messenger to His people. Isaiah saw the Lord Himself sitting on a lofty throne with the train of His robe filling the Temple. Hovering around Him were a mighty chorus of angels singing, "Holy, holy, holy is the Lord Almighty! The whole earth is filled with His glory!" Their glorious singing shook the Temple to its foundations, filling the entire sanctuary with smoke. Isaiah was awestruck by God's greatness and power compared to his own sinfulness: "My destruction is sealed, for I am a sinful man and a member of a sinful race. Yet I have seen the King, the Lord Almighty!" He came to fully understand the extent of God's forgiveness as one of the angels touched his lips with a burning coal, removing his guilt, forgiving his sins, and giving him the power to do God's work (Isaiah 6:1-7).

The burning coal represents the painful cleansing process

many of God's servants go through before accepting and fulfilling His call in their lives. Moses lived isolated and alone in the desert for 40 years before God called him to rescue the Israelites from Egypt. Joseph was sold into slavery by his own brothers and imprisoned for 13 years before he became the ruler of Egypt and saved Israel from starvation. David spent years hiding in caves and running for his life before he became king. For many of us today, broken relationships, addictions, losses, and other life crises can drive us to the pit of despair before we realize our need for God and how we might be called to serve Him. Cancer was my burning coal. It brought me into His throne room and helped me understand my own sin and brokenness before a pure and holy God. Cancer taught me how desperately I needed a Savior and how powerless I was to do anything of lasting value without Him. Before I could accept God's call to write, speak or do anything else for Him — before I could minister to the hurting — I needed to be cleansed and forgiven so I could fully submit to His control.

When God asked, "Who will go?" Isaiah submitted himself fully to His service. God didn't force His will on Isaiah; he heard God's call and responded freely. He had seen the face of God and was humbled by His grace and mercy. Perhaps cancer brought you to the throne room where you, too, had a personal encounter with the Lord. Perhaps it was your burning coal. Have you heard Him asking? "Whom should I send as a messenger to my people? Who will go?" Submit to Him freely, and God will send you into the world to share His wonderful message of hope with the hurting and discouraged (2 Corinthians 5:18-20). After all, you've cried their tears. You've felt their pain. You've experienced His grace and mercy. When He asks, will your answer be the same? "Lord, I'll go! Send me."

Father, your glory and majesty overwhelm me. I want to see your face and understand the full extent of your grace and mercy. When I hear your call, help me to answer, "Send me!" Amen.

16

The Light That Leads to Life

For you have rescued me from death; you have kept my feet from slipping. So now, I can walk in your presence God, in your life-giving light. — Psalm 56:13

There was something about Halloween that always delighted our children. Maybe it was seeing who could carve the scariest pumpkin or planning for months what creepy creature they would be for Halloween. Maybe it was just the candy. When the spooky night finally arrived, they joined all the other little ghosts and goblins for a night of trick or treating through the dark streets of our neighborhood. The "best" houses were always decked out with crooked grave markers etched with R.I.P., zombies rising out of coffins, and dimly lit porches draped with bats and cobwebs. The kids would ring the doorbell and collect their treat from some ghoulish homeowner to the sounds of howling wind, groans, and blood curdling screams. Maybe all the fun was in the pretending. They could dip their toes in a little doom and gloom and let themselves get frightened, but they always knew mom and dad were right behind them with the flashlight.

Darkness often conjures up thoughts of despair, death, and gloom. Sometimes cancer feels that way, only with cancer, there is no pretending. Sometimes, it can feel like a nightmare that never ends. You wonder if the checkups, statistics, and memories will hold you captive under a dark cloud of uncertainty forever. But Jesus came as a light to shine into your nightmare (John 12:46). Darkness can never extinguish light and evil cannot and will not overcome the light of God (John 1:4-5).

Once when Jesus was teaching in the part of the Temple where candles burned to symbolize the pillar of fire that led the Israelites through the wilderness, He said to the people: "I am the light of the world. If you follow me, you won't be stumbling through the darkness, because you will have the light that leads to life" (John 8:12). The pillar of fire was the presence of Almighty God. The same light that guided the Israelites through the wilderness to the Promised Land is still available for you today. The light of His presence will protect and lead you safely through the darkest fears and doubts.

Praise God, for He has rescued you from death and kept your feet from slipping! When the darkness creeps in unexpectedly and evil thoughts of death and despair threaten to tell you otherwise, remember that your heavenly Daddy is always behind you with His flashlight. Take some time everyday to bask in His life-giving light. He is the fountain of life, the light by which you see (Psalm 36:9). He will light the path ahead of you and you will never stumble into the dark corners of fear and uncertainty again. Walk in His presence to a future of hope and new beginnings. He is the light the leads to life.

Father, thank you for being the life-giving light that rescued me from death. Please lead me safely through my darkest fears and doubts into a future of hope and certainty in you. Amen.

17

It is Well

Dear friend, I am praying that all is well with you and that your body is as healthy as I know your soul is. — 3 John 1:2

Everyone has a packed schedule, a bad day a work, or a friend or family member that disappoints. Have you ever noticed that these times of stress and emotional upheaval often lead to physical symptoms? Maybe it's a migraine headache or a cold that seems to come on at the worst possible time. When the season of discontent is extended and the anxiety mounts, the physical manifestation can be more serious. Years ago, my cancer diagnosis came after a long period of unbridled emotional stress. Coincidence? Maybe, but I don't think so.

The soul is the part of us that encompasses our mind, will, and emotions. When David was pursued by his enemies and then rejected by his friends, he described a strong connection between the body and soul: "Have mercy on me Lord for I am in distress. My sight is blurred because of my tears. My body and soul are withering away. I am dying from grief; my years are shortened by sadness. Misery has drained my strength. I am wasting away from within" (Psalm 31:9-10). Not only did emotional distress impact his body, but it threatened to take years off his life.

We can't always control the circumstances around us, but we can strive to keep our soul healthy in the midst of them. A healthy soul seeks to know God, is open to His nature, and seeks to be in a right relationship with Him. David's soul was in anguish but he continued to trust God's provision, unfailing love, and faithfulness. He believed in the goodness of God in spite of the gravity of his situation (Psalm 31:7-8, 19-20). He knew only God could fully satisfy his thirst in the parched and weary condition he found himself in (Psalm 63:1).

Horatio G. Spafford wrote the famous hymn, "It Is Well With My Soul" after two major traumas in his life. The great Chicago Fire of October 1871 ruined him financially and shortly after, all four of his daughters died in a collision with another ship while crossing the Atlantic. Several weeks later as his own ship passed near the spot where his daughters died, the Holy Spirit inspired these words:

> *When peace, like a river, attendeth my way,*
> *When sorrows like sea billows roll;*
> *Whatever my lot, Thou has taught me to say,*
> *It is well, it is well, with my soul.*

A healthy soul has an eternal hope anchored in Christ. The Apostle John knew his friend's soul was healthy because he was faithful and living in the truth (3 John 1:3). His selfless service to Christ's church reflected his obedience to the ways of God. I pray you too will have a healthy soul that hungers for God and hears His voice. May His truth penetrate deep into your heart and bring you radiant health (Proverbs 4:21-22). May your steadfast obedience to Him lead to a long and good life (Proverbs 4:10). And may you always be able to say, regardless of the stress and strain life brings, "it is well, it is well, with my soul."

Father, thank you for your provision, your unfailing love, and your faithfulness, even when I don't understand my circumstances. Help me anchor my soul in you, Jesus. It is well. Amen.

18

KINGDOM LIVING

The thief's purpose is to steal and kill and destroy. My purpose is to give life in all its fullness. — John 10:10

When I speak, I like to give my testimony and share how God healed me from breast cancer. It always raises a few eyebrows when I tell them God did not give me cancer and it was not His will that I should suffer from it. While God often gets the blame when bad things happen, it's Satan the thief whose purpose it is to steal, kill, and destroy. Jesus, on the other hand, came to give His followers a life of abundance. When He walked the face of this earth, He didn't go around inflicting people with disease and calamity. He healed and delivered them (Acts 10:36-38). A woman challenged me once and told me that the promise of John 10:10 is not for us believers today, but only for us when we die and go to Heaven. Really?

Cancer, chemo, and a lifetime of fear were never God's plan for you. In fact, He has plans for good and not disaster. He came to give you a future and a hope (Jeremiah 29:11). Your eternal future started the moment you received Jesus as your Lord and Savior. His precious gift at Calvary bought you so much more than a ticket to Heaven when you die someday. The Good News Jesus preached in Matthew 4:17 and throughout the Gospels is that the

Kingdom of Heaven is near! He didn't just go around announcing the Good News of the Kingdom. He demonstrated it. As the news about Jesus spread, people began bringing to Him all who were sick. And whatever their sickness or disease, or if they were demon possessed or epileptic or paralyzed — He healed them all (Matthew 4:23-24).

Heaven touched earth when Jesus came. He brought with Him the Kingdom of God, and He is the same yesterday, today, and forever (Hebrews 13:8). He never changes. The Kingdom is not just a future place, but a realm of real power that exists today where people are healed, lives are restored, and miracles happen. When we live in the Kingdom under God's rule and reign, by the power of the Holy Spirit, there is love, joy, peace, goodness, and abundant life. How many times have you prayed the words, "thy Kingdom come, thy will be done on earth as it is in Heaven?" His Kingdom has come and there is no cancer in Heaven.

If you believe your cancer came from God, it might have been difficult to ask Him for healing. And you might struggle to believe that staying cancer free is also God's will. Yes, God can and will use your suffering for His glory and purposes, but that doesn't mean He willed it to happen. It's difficult to trust God for something you believe is contrary to His plan for your life. But Jesus said if you have seen Him, you have seen His Father. If you want to know how God feels about you, just study the life of His Son. He overflowed with love and compassion. Every person who came to Him left healed and free. And He wants the same for you. Seek His Kingdom in all you do and begin walking in the abundant life He planned for you all along. You may come back to earth to visit once in awhile, but I guarantee, you won't stay long.

Father, thank you for the abundant life you won for me on the cross. Show me how to live in the fullness of your Kingdom today. Amen.

19

The Way of Life

You will show me the way of life, granting me the joy of your presence and the pleasures of living with you forever. — Psalm 16:11

Imagine yourself on a long journey to a far away destination. You have the trip mapped out to the best of your knowledge, but before you are barely on your way, you reach a fork in the road. This Y-intersection doesn't show up on your map and your GPS has no explanation. Marking the road going to the right is a sign that reads, "The Way of Life." The sign marking the road to the left reads, "The Way of Death." Which road do you take? It's a safe bet you'll be making a right turn.

This seems like such an obvious choice, yet so often on the journey through life after cancer we find ourselves veering left and getting lost in the land of worries and what ifs. By the time the next dreaded appointment comes and we have spent every waking hour on the Internet looking for evidence of the possibilities we fear most, the enemy has created in us a false and distorted reality. When we worry about tomorrow and fear what might happen, we are projecting future events without including God in the image we have conjured up in our minds. The Lord said that people who put their trust in mere humans and turn their hearts away from

Him are like stunted shrubs in the desert, with no hope for the future. They will live in the barren wilderness, on the salty flats where no one lives (Jeremiah 17:5-6). We veer left on that fork in the road and this is the scenery we'll find. There is no joy or pleasure in living this way.

On the other hand, if you choose the way of life, His powerful presence will lead you along the path of righteousness and to all the good things He has in store for you. Your health is a blessing and the Source of all blessings promises to guard it along with everything else that belongs to you (Psalm 16:2, 5). Stay on this road under His protective wing and you will not be shaken, regardless of the circumstances that threaten to steal your joy. He is right beside you and your body rests in safety (Psalm 16:8-9). Instead of stunted shrubs in the desert, those who travel the way of life are like trees planted along riverbanks with roots that reach deep into the water. They are not bothered by the heat or long months of drought. Their leaves stay green, and they go right on producing delicious fruit (Jeremiah 17: 7-8).

In your journey through life after cancer, you may reach this fork in the road several times a day. Problems may come, circumstances may distract you, and fear and worry may try to pull you to the left. You can stay on course by keeping your eyes focused on Jesus, the author and finisher of your faith (Hebrews 12:2). Let His Spirit guide you into all truth and reveal to you whatever you need to know. Allow His Word to instruct and correct you and prepare you for every good thing He wants you to do (2 Timothy 3:16-17). Every day, let Him show you the way of life. Then bask in the joy of His presence and experience the pleasures of living with Him forever.

Father, thank you for leading me along the path of righteousness and to all the good things you have in store for me. Help me to stay on course and to keep my eyes on the way of life. Amen.

20

His Place of Rest

For this Good News – that God has prepared a place of rest — has been announced to us just as it was to them. But it did them no good because they didn't believe what God told them. For only we who believe can enter his place of rest. — Hebrews 4:2-3

The Israelites had finally arrived. God led them out of slavery, through the desolate wilderness, and to the very edge of the rich and fertile land He had promised to give their ancestors. Throughout the journey, He guided them, fed them, protected them, performed amazing miracles, and fulfilled all His promises. Now, as a final step before entering the Promised Land, He commanded Moses to send twelve scouts to explore it (Numbers 13:1-20). They returned forty days later with a conflicting report. It truly was a magnificent country, a land flowing with milk and honey. But it was inhabited by a powerful people living in large and fortified cities, and giants so large that the Israelites felt like grasshoppers next to them (Numbers 13:25-33).

Two scouts, Caleb and Joshua, encouraged the people to not be afraid and to trust God's promise to bring them safely home (Numbers 14:6-9). But the people refused, even though reaching the Promised Land had been their goal since leaving Egypt. As a result of their unbelief, they wandered the desert for forty years until an entire generation died. Only Joshua and Caleb would enter the land because they trusted God would do what He promised (Numbers 14:20-34).

Your promised land is not the land of Canaan where Joshua would eventually lead the Israelites, but a new place of rest prepared just for you (Hebrews 4:6-10). It is a place we enter through faith in Christ. It is both an eternal rest we receive on a new earth to come, and a peace we receive today by trusting and obeying Him. It is found in the throne room of God where we can boldly enter and receive His grace and mercy (Hebrews 4:14-16). As a child of God, the same promises God gave to Abraham belong to you (Galatians 3:29). When you walk in His ways, He promises to bless you wherever you go, bless everything you do, and to conquer your enemies when they attack you. He promises to provide for you from his rich treasury in the heavens and give you an abundance of good things in the land he is giving you (Deuteronomy 28:1-14).

Have you arrived in your promised land or are you lingering around the border? Sometimes, like the Israelites, we can fail to enter our place of rest. Even though the treatment is over, the hair has grown back, and we know God's Word says we have been healed by His stripes, we stand on the edge of the promise and still live and think like someone with cancer. We wander in the wilderness of doubt and uncertainty instead of receiving God's promises of healing, provision, and the abundance of good things that wait for us in our promised land. His promises did the Israelites no good because they didn't believe what God told them. Don't make this same mistake. Step out in faith and receive what belongs to you. Because only we who believe can enter his place of rest.

Father, thank for the abundance of good things that wait for me in my promised land. I don't want to wander in a wilderness of doubt and uncertainty. Help me to trust you and enter your place of rest. Amen.

21

GOD ENCOUNTER

May you experience the love of Christ, though it is so great you will never fully understand it. Then you will be filled with the fullness of life and power that comes from God. — Ephesians 3:19

If you ever went to Sunday school and sang "Jesus Loves Me" or watched a Billy Graham crusade on television, you know God loves you. But what does it mean to experience His love? After cancer, I grew more desperate to know this God who healed me. The Bible says we are to worship Him in Spirit and in truth (John 4:23-24). A devoted Bible reader, I knew God loved me and had good things planned for my life. I knew He would provide for my every need. But as the months passed, I hungered to experience the truth I read about in the Bible, to see all God's promises become real in my life and in the lives of others, and live in the fullness of His power within me. He healed me of cancer and I was so grateful. But I wanted everything God had in store for me. I wanted all of Him. So I began to pray for more.

One day at a conference, I went to the front to receive prayer. I was deeply moved by a teaching on the Father's love, and the presence of the Holy Spirit was powerful. I looked to my right, and to my surprise, people were falling on the floor like dominoes as the pastor prayed for them. I wanted to run, but something kept my feet firmly planted. As the pastor approached me, I prayed, "God if this is you, you have to show me now." As the pastor laid his hands on me and began to pray, God poured out His love with such power that my knees buckled and I found myself flat on my back on the floor along with everyone else around me. I don't know how long I laid there. It could have been minutes or hours, it didn't really matter. All I remember is resting in the joy of His presence, being overwhelmed by His peace and held captive by His love. I could have stayed there forever. I experienced the love of Christ that day, but I know there is so much more. His love is so great, our human minds can't begin to comprehend it. I realized that day I would spend the rest of my life and all of eternity discovering the width, the length, the height, and the depth of God's love (Ephesians 3:18).

I'm learning that encountering God is much more than reading about Him in the Bible and knowing about Him in my head. Experiencing the Scripture through the power of the Holy Spirit makes it come alive and become real in my life. The Word says God loves me with an everlasting love and with this unfailing love, He draws me to Himself (Jeremiah 31:3). But until I began to receive and experience it, His love was head knowledge, not heart knowledge.

The more you know and experience God's love, the more you will walk in the fullness of Christ. He can fill every aspect of your life to the fullest with His light, love, wisdom, holiness, power, and glory. He completes you. Pray for a God encounter today. Pray to experience His love, though it is so great you will never fully understand it. Then you will be filled with the fullness of life and power that only comes from God.

Father, thank you for your presence, your power, and for loving me with an everlasting love. Help me to step out of my comfort zone and experience all that you have for me. I want more! Amen.

22

STAND FIRM

Put on all of God's armor so that you will be able to stand firm against all strategies and tricks of the Devil. — Ephesians 6:11

I woke up today knowing my schedule for the morning included a mammogram and a check up at the Breast Center. Even though it's been several years since I was diagnosed and the cancer never showed up in a mammogram anyway, there was a tiny part of me that wanted to stay in bed. Strange, because I know I'm healed. I don't spend one minute of time worried that I'm not. But there's something about this particular appointment at this particular clinic that conjures up old memories. Maybe it's the familiar smell when the elevator opens to the 4th floor or the fact that the oncologist's office where I received eight rounds of chemo is located right next door to the Breast Center. In any case, they are memories I'd rather forget.

I normally pray when I wake up, and this morning was no different. But on this morning, I spent some extra time praying God's supernatural armor over myself. I've learned that Satan lurks in the bushes waiting to attack at moments like this (1 Peter 5:6). All he needs is a tiny little crack in the armor to gain a foothold into my soul and stir up feelings of doubt and fear. This particular morning, he didn't have a chance.

I started by putting on my helmet of salvation to protect my mind from doubting God's saving work in my life (Ephesians 6:17). I thanked Him for the precious gift of His Son who conquered the fear of death and gave me an abundant life and an eternal destiny (Hebrews 2:15; John 10:10). Next, I put on the breastplate of righteousness to protect my heart when Satan tries to make me feel unworthy and unaccepted (Ephesians 6:14). I thanked Him that I am made holy by the blood of His Son (2 Corinthians 5:21). His belt of truth helps me to discern and defeat Satan's lies and keeps me firmly focused on His promise that I have been healed by His stripes. The shoes of peace give me the courage to confidently walk into enemy territory and proclaim the true peace found only in God. I hold up the shield of faith to stop every fiery arrow the enemy throws at me (Ephesians 6:14-16).

Finally, I take the sword of the Spirit, God's Word, and use it the same way Jesus used it on the Devil during his forty days in the wilderness (Ephesians 6:17; Matthew 4:1-11). By knowing and receiving God's Word into my heart, I can speak it out loud in the power of the Spirit and by the authority of Jesus to counter the enemy's lies. By the time my feet hit the floor, the enemy's plan had been thwarted.

Will he ever give us a rest? No, Satan's goal is to advance his kingdom and extend his sphere of influence (Ephesians 2:2; 2 Corinthians 4:4). In your journey through life, he will look for many opportunities to lie, cheat, and steal your destiny. He wants you to doubt your God, doubt your healing, and fear for your future. His primary tactic is to use these tricks to distract you from pure and sincere devotion to Christ (2 Corinthians 11:3). But God didn't leave you defenseless in your battle against doubt and fear.

Even though the enemy will try to convince you otherwise, Jesus already defeated him. In Christ, you are assured of ultimate victory (Romans 8:37). So resist the devil and he will flee from you (James 4:7). Put on all of God's armor so you are able to stand firm.

Father, thank you for the ultimate victory I have in Christ and the spiritual armor that protects me from the enemy's attacks. Help me to proclaim your truth and stand firm. Amen.

23

IF THE LORD WANTS

How do you know what your life will be like tomorrow?
Your life is like the morning fog — it's here a little while, then it's
gone. What you ought to say is, "If the Lord wants us to, we will live
and do this or that." Otherwise you are boasting about your own
plans, and all such boasting is evil. — James 4:14-16

No one really wants to hang around Minnesota in January unless they enjoy 30 consecutive days of sub-zero temperatures, snow shoveling, and 14-foot snow drifts. Our jobs allow us to work and travel out of our home, so one day it occurred to us … maybe we could work from someplace else in January; someplace a lot warmer than Minnesota. Maybe we could work from Florida. We took the plunge and rented a house on Sanibel Island just to get a taste of what it was like to join the other "snowbirds" who bailed on Minnesota in the dead of winter. We counted the months until our great adventure. Finally, a few days after Christmas when the cold and snow had everyone else locked inside for another season of cabin fever, we packed up and headed south.

The house was beautiful; three bedrooms to accommodate visits from family and friends, a caged pool and spa to keep the bugs and alligators away, and only a short bike ride to the beach. It was a perfect plan except for one small detail; we froze. We didn't just encounter record breaking lows. We encountered record setting lows. Who ever heard of temperatures in the twenties and thirties on Sanibel Island? For at least two weeks, it was even too cold to enjoy the heated pool in the sunshine. But I wasn't just cold. I was mad. I was mad until one evening while sitting on the beach bundled up in my winter coat, I watched the most stunning sunset I had ever seen in my life. God finally got my attention.

You see, it's not about the weather. It's not about my basking in the sun by the swimming pool while everyone else is home freezing in Minnesota. It's all about God. I forget sometimes. I forget that it's not about me and my elaborate plans. It's about the one that healed me and makes me whole, the one who completes me. In Him, I live and breathe and have my very being (Acts 28:17). He is sovereign over my very existence. Without His grace, there would be no trips to Florida, no plans or dreams to look forward to, no life to celebrate or family and friends to celebrate with. Without Him, I am nothing.

This is a humbling thought for most of us. We live under the delusion that it's all about us. And we like to think that somehow on this road through life, we have control over the road map. In our pride and frustration, we often push God out of the driver's seat and take over the wheel. Yes, we can and should make plans, but we need to do so while holding on loosely to the things of this world. God's ways are higher than ours and His plans are always better, even when we don't understand them at the time (Isaiah 55:8-9). He didn't just heal me so I could go to Florida and bask in the sunshine, although I know it gives Him great joy to give me the desires of my heart. He didn't even heal me so I could serve Him.

He healed me simply because He loves me. And I learned years ago that basking in the light of His love is better than life itself. I want to live with that reality all the days of my life.

Never forget that you are not your own; you were bought at a price (1 Corinthians 6:19-10). He didn't save you to live for yourself but to honor Him (Romans 14:7-8). We really can't be certain about what tomorrow may bring or the weather in Florida, but we can always be certain of God. And God wants to bless you infinitely more than you would ever dare to ask or hope (Ephesians 3:20). Trust that He loves you and wants the very best for you. As you bask in His glory today, pray that the desires of His heart become the desires of yours. Then go ahead and make your plans. If the Lord wants, maybe I'll see you in Florida sometime.

Father, thank you for your grace and for making me whole. I know you always want the very best for me. Forgive me when I take over the wheel and forget who's in the driver seat. Amen.

24

MEMORY STONES

When all the people had crossed the Jordan, the LORD said to Joshua, "Now choose twelve men, one from each tribe. Tell them, 'Take twelve stones from the very place where the priests are standing in the middle of the Jordan. Carry them out and pile them up at the place where you will camp tonight.'" — Joshua 4:1

The third Monday of every month, I go back. I've been going back to that same dark pit every since God rescued me from it. It was never my plan to go back. It was His. Shortly after my treatment ended, I founded Pray for the Cure, a healing and discipleship ministry for people struggling with all types of cancer. In addition to our regular monthly prayer meetings, the ministry has taken me to the bedside of people in hospitals and hospices, and to special appointments in the prayer chapel and private homes to deliver God's message of hope and offer healing prayer to the sick and hurting.

When I go back into battle against the same enemy who tried to steal my health and my future, I feel God's anointing and protection on me. I feel His call on my life to bless and pray for others caught in the same pit He rescued me from. Best of all, I remember what God did for me. I remember how He has poured His blessing on my life. I remember His faithfulness and miraculous healing power and how He comforted me when I was in the same dark pit. I remember the way I felt in His presence and how desperate I am for more of Him. I'm reminded that I never want to go back to my old life because He is more than enough. Pray for the Cure is one of my "memory stones."

Memory stones are important reminders of God's faithfulness as we establish our own personal history with God. There are numerous accounts in the Bible of how the Israelites built memorials to forever remind them of God's goodness and miraculous power. For example:

• God directed Joshua to build a memorial from 12 stones drawn from the river by 12 men from each tribe to remind the people that God guided them across the Jordan on dry ground (Joshua 4:1-9).

• After Jacob awoke from the dream where God offered him the same covenant promise He had made to Abraham and Isaac, Jacob took the stone he had used as his pillow and set it upright as a memorial pillar to mark a place for worshipping God (Genesis 28:18-22).

• After the LORD helped the Israelites defeat the Philistine army, Samuel set up a larger stone and named it Ebenezer, or the "stone of help," and said, "Up to this point, the LORD has helped us" (1 Samuel 7:12).

Moses impressed on the Israelites to repeat God's commands again and again to their children, to tie them to their hands as a reminder, and to wear them on the doorposts of their houses and on their gates. Then he said when the children asked about the meaning of these commands, they would be able to tell how the Lord brought them out of Egypt with amazing power (Deuteronomy 6:7-8; 20-21). Where are you building memorials to God's faithfulness and power in your life? What is your Pray for the Cure? Many people keep a journal and then go back to read their stories of victory when they need reassurance of God's faithfulness. I mark up my Bible with dates, places, events, and comments in the margins. Not only am I reminded of God's blessings at particular times in my life every time I open my Bible, but I have a wonderful heritage to pass on to my children. Yes, He is God and He is faithful. He was, He is, and always will be your Comforter, Helper, and Healer. Pile up those memory stones today and let them be an ongoing testimony of His power and love.

Father, thank you that I can be a testimony of your blessing and protection in the lives of others. Help me to build a visible memorial to your faithfulness and power. Amen.

25

HAND OF VICTORY

Don't be afraid, for I am with you. Don't be discouraged,
for I am your God. I will strengthen you and help you. I will hold
you up with my victorious right hand. — Isaiah 41: 41:10

I can't count the times a cancer survivor has confided in me days or hours before a routine check up with the oncologist. I've seen shaking, tears, white knuckles, and even skin rashes at the thought of returning to the clinic for these routine tests. At the beginning of this book, I shared a comment from a reader who described how the thought of another scan sends her to her knees and how she waits in paralyzing fear for the cancer to come back and steal the rest of her life.

I've often wondered if the doctors and nurses who work in these clinics really know how their well intended words and actions impact cancer survivors. Instead of assuming health and healing, these vigilant healthcare workers often approach these visits as though their patients still have cancer, even when it isn't clinically present. No wonder these visits conjure up so much fear and trepidation.

When battling this fear, we can learn much from King David. Even though David was anointed future king, he spent many years hiding in caves while running from King Saul and fearing for his life. The Psalms express his feelings during this time and how he coped. Like many cancer survivors, David described his fear as paralyzing and a threat to his hope (Psalm 143:4). He pleaded with God to hear and answer his cries for help (Psalm 143:1). Then he trusted God to conquer his fear: "Though a mighty army surrounds me, my heart will know no fear. Even if they attack me, I remain confident" (Psalm 27:3).

If you are struggling with fear today, you need to know it is not from God. God didn't give you a spirit of fear and timidity, but of power, love, and self-discipline (2 Timothy 1:7). When fear threatens to overwhelm you, know that it is a lie from the pit of hell. God warns us to be careful and watch out for attacks from the Devil who prowls around like a roaring lion, looking for some victim to devour (1 Peter 5:8). And there is no more likely victim than a cancer survivor heading to the oncologist's office for a routine checkup.

The good news is that you never have to face fear alone. God is with you. He was with David in the caves and freed him from all his fears (Psalm 34:4). His Son Jesus assured the disciples of His presence in the middle of the lake when the storm raged around them and they screamed in terror thinking He was a ghost. "Don't be afraid, He said. "Take courage, I am here" (Mark 6:50)! His Holy Spirit living inside us brings a deep and lasting supernatural peace and the confident assurance that we have no need to fear the present or the future (John 14:27). So when fear rises up, His response is always the same: Don't be afraid. I am with you wherever you go (Joshua 1:9). From this check up to the next, from this day and beyond, I will hold you up in my victorious right hand.

Father, thank you for your calming presence that is with me wherever I go. Help me, God! Hold me high above my fears in your right hand of victory. Amen.

26

THE ONE WHO MAKES THE PROMISE

*Then Jesus said to the disciples, "Have faith in God. I tell you
the truth, you can say to this mountain, 'May you be lifted up and
thrown into the sea,' and it will happen. But you must really believe
it will happen and have no doubt in your heart. I tell you,
you can pray for anything, and if you believe that you've received it,
it will be yours."* — Mark 11:22-24

My husband has logged over 75,000 miles on our Gold Wing
touring motorcycle, and most of those miles with me on the back
seat. Sometimes the destination is across the country and sometimes
it's across town. Everyone knows the dangers of motorcycling. We're
safety conscious and wear helmets and leathers for protection.
When the weather cooperates, we enjoy riding the open roads and
basking in God's beautiful creation under sunny skies. On days
like this, the leathers usually come off. But sometimes the weather
doesn't cooperate. Sometimes, especially on long trips, we've been
caught on the open road with no option but to keep going until
the next meal or the next gas stop. My husband says that's why God
created rain suits, chaps, and heated gear.

Through all this, I've learned that when he says we're going
to arrive safely in Duluth before dinner, I believe what he says.

I believe what he says because I trust him. He is a seasoned motorcyclist with precious cargo in the back. I can trust him because I'm in an intimate relationship with him. He loves me and we communicate about such things. Something occurred to me one day while speeding down the freeway at 70 miles per hour in blistering hot weather with big semi trucks passing on my right and left — if I can trust my husband to get me safely to Duluth in these conditions, I can certainly trust the Creator of the Universe to move my mountain.

Jesus says if you command your mountain to be lifted up and thrown into the sea, it will happen if you really believe it will happen and have no doubt in your heart. But He also tells us that the first requirement to believing is to have faith in God. In order to believe the promise and have no doubt, I have to fully trust the one who made the promise. I have to hear His voice, seek His face, and know He is real. I have to encounter Him and experience Him personally. I could never trust my life on the back of the Gold Wing to a driver I didn't know intimately. His promises would ring hollow.

Do you truly know the one who makes the promise? The one healed you by His stripes, released the captives, and freed the downtrodden from their oppressors (Isaiah 53:4; Luke 4:18)? The one who gives beauty for ashes, joy instead of mourning, and praise instead of despair (Isaiah 61:3)? He's inviting you into a personal relationship today. He is more than the Savior who died for your sins. He is your companion, your soul mate and your very best friend. Ask Him for more; more of His love, more His power, and more His presence. Seek to hear His voice and seek His face. As you grow in intimacy with Him, you will grow in your capacity to pray for anything and believe His Word. And if you believe that you've already received it, it will be yours.

Father, thank you for your Son, my Savior. I want more! I want to fully trust you, Lord. Show me who you really are. Amen.

27

THE ART OF WAITING

In quietness and confidence is your strength. — Isaiah 30:15

What are you waiting for? Life after cancer brings a whole new meaning to an age old question. Before, you may have been waiting for the right time to change jobs, to move, to marry, to take up a new hobby, to join a church, or to go back to school. Maybe you were waiting for God to answer a specific prayer for yourself or a loved one, or to bring clarity to an area of confusion in your life. Now, you find yourself waiting for life to just be normal again, for the doctor to confirm you are well (again), for the dark cloud of uncertainty to lift, and to see a clear, certain pathway ahead for the rest of your life. Perhaps you are waiting for strength to face each new day and confidence that the Lord will help you embrace your future with renewed hope and expectation.

The true answer to this question lies in the silence — the still and quiet times you spend waiting before the Lord. These are not the times we bring before Him our list of petitions, or the worldly interests, concerns, and fears that occupy our minds. It's not even a time for Bible reading, prayerful thoughts, or to bring before Him the deepest hopes, desires, and dreams that engage our hearts. It is a time to completely separate ourselves from family and friends, work and leisure, joys and sorrows, all the things of the world — even all the things of God — to be truly quiet before Him. In true waiting, your whole heart is turned toward God and there is nothing on your mind but God Himself.

To fully grasp what it means to wait on the Lord, imagine if the physical presence of God Himself manifested in front of you. Imagine meeting Him face to face. What will you do? When God appeared before Moses in the form of a burning bush, he hid is face in his hands (Exodus 3:6). Later, when bringing the disobedience of the people before the Lord, he fell facedown and laid prostrate before Him for forty days and forty nights (Deuteronomy 9:25). Zechariah was overwhelmed with fear at God's presence (Luke 1:12). At the transfiguration, Peter, John, and James fell face down to the ground at the presence of God (Matthew 17:6). Even if you don't fall face down to the ground, the very thought of coming into the sovereign, majestic presence of God should silence your heart and mind. It is no wonder that the prophet Habakkuk exclaimed "Let all the earth keep silence before Him" (Habakkuk 2:20)!

My daughter has a big stuffed pillow and a little lamp on a stand in the corner of her walk in closet where she plays soft worship music and connects with God. She calls it her "prayer closet." When you set aside time in your own prayer closet to truly wait on God with no strings attached, you receive a priceless gift. You may not receive the answer to prayer you so desperately covet, or even a better prayer life. As your humble soul waits in the holy stillness, you receive the unspeakable blessing of God Himself. No answers, no directions, just God. He meets you face to face in this sacred place. He reveals Himself. He speaks to you. And you may have no choice but to lay prostrate before Him. You know that He alone will do His wondrous work in your life, whatever the future might bring. In quietness and confidence, your strength comes.

Father, thank you for the silence of your presence. Help me to wait in your holy stillness with no strings attached. Amen.

28

The Matter is Closed

"I also tell you this: If two of you agree here on earth concerning anything you ask, my Father in heaven will do it for you. For where two or three gather together as my followers, I am there among them."
— Matthew 18:19-20

Time is my friend. As the weeks, months, and years pass by, I think less and less about cancer, all the unpleasant ways it disrupted my life, and how it threatened to steal my future. In fact, other than living with a full and grateful heart for all God has done in my life, I can literally go for weeks without thinking about it at all. I don't think God remembers it either. He doesn't remember the cancer that attacked my body anymore than He remembers the sin that threatened to steal my soul. He conquered them both. In one single sacrificial act, He removed the power of sin forever (Hebrews 9:26). When He deals with our sin and all its destructive powers, He separates it from us as far as the east is from the west and doesn't give it another thought (Psalm 103:12). And neither should we.

As much as I want the dark side of cancer to be permanently erased from my brain, there are always a few people who believe it's their call and duty in life to help me remember. I had an encounter with one of these concerned and well-meaning individuals one

Sunday after church, about ten years after I was diagnosed. She was a former neighbor, a prominent woman in our community who I hadn't seen in several years. As I was leaving church, she was coming in and locked eyes with me in the entry way. With deep sadness and pity in her eyes, she gushed, "Oh my, how are you doing dear?" Her head shook slowly back and forth and the foreboding look on her face was of someone paying respects to a dying friend. I can't count how many times over the years I've had to explain to people that "I'm fine" and that "God healed me." I went through that same ritual again, smiled, thanked her for her concern, and told her to have a blessed day. My husband immediately put his arm around me and whispered a prayer in my ear, rebuking her words and any power they might have on me.

She meant well. There are still those who believe cancer and other serious illnesses are automatic death sentences, and it's just a matter of time. They're still bracing themselves for the bad news, and surprised to see you out and about, living an active, normal, healthy life. It disrupts their paradigm and you can see the confusion in their faces. They may be wonderful people, but they are not an encouragement to you. They are part of a world that is not in agreement with your healing, and you should avoid receiving their words like the plague. They want to remind you of something God has already forgotten. In essence, they are coming into agreement with the enemy, the author of death and disease.

I'm grateful my husband was with me that day and that I have surrounded myself with believing brothers and sisters in Christ who are in agreement with the healing work of Jesus in my life. Ecclesiastics 4:12 reminds us that a person standing alone can be attacked and defeated, but two can stand back-to-back and conquer.

If you are separate from other believing Christians, encountering inevitable people or situations that challenge your health status will stir up fear and doubt. Jesus said if you and two or more agree concerning anything that lines up with His Word, He is in the midst of that agreement to see that it comes to pass. Any attempts to conjure up the past and bring your cancer back to life do not come from God. As far as He's concerned, the matter is closed.

Father, thank you for removing the power of sin from my life and forgetting my past. Please surround me with people who agree with the healing work of Christ in all areas of my life. Amen.

29

STINKIN' THINKIN'

Don't copy the behavior and customs of this world, but let God transform you into a new person by changing the way you think. Then you will learn to know God's will for you, which is good and pleasing and perfect. — Romans 12:2

Let's face it. Living in this world doesn't always bring good thoughts to our minds. To anyone who doubts the existence of Satan, I say look around you. Just watching the nightly news or reading the newspaper points to the selfishness and corruption that dominates our local, national and international scene. The latest movies or even the latest prime time TV line up gives a snapshot of the degradation of society. Evil pervades the world we live in, sometimes in the most subtle places. Even Christians can sometimes be prideful, stubborn, covetous, and selfish. As a cancer survivor, you have intimately experienced the work of the enemy and the thinking of the world. That evil can continue to rear its ugly head through anyone or anything that tempts you to believe your healing isn't real. Several years ago, a doctor said to me, "Sooner or later, this cancer will get you." Her comment reflected worldly thinking, did not align with God's will, and certainly wasn't "good and pleasing and perfect."

In your quest for health and freedom, you can be tempted to allow the behaviors, customs, words, and mindsets of this world to bring you down. You can let "stinkin' thinkin'" consume you and wallow in self-pity, anxiety, confusion, or doubt. Or, you can let God transform you into a new person by changing the way you think. One of the best ways to allow God to change your thinking is through "declarative prayer." In this type of prayer, instead of making requests of God, you come to Him in prayer and declare His truth. Declarative prayer is not a substitute for petitioning God, but another way to pray, especially when your spirits are down, you are barraged by ungodly messages, tempted by unbelief, and consumed by stinkin' thinkin'. It lifts you out of the pit, changes your mindsets, reorients your thinking, and increases faith.

Declarative prayer starts by giving God permission to access your mind. Pray that He would hold all your thoughts, both good and bad, captive under the authority of Jesus (2 Corinthians 10: 4-5). Then, let your thoughts take the form of words that you speak out loud in faith. These words might come directly from Scripture or they may be words that God speaks directly to your spirit. In either case, speaking out the promises of God interrupts the facts, reality, and lies that surround you and brings the truth of God into your situation. The more you declare what He says, the more you believe it.

A good example of declarative prayer is Psalm 23. David doesn't ask God to be his shepherd; he declares that God is. He doesn't ask God to meet his needs; He declares that God will. Throughout the psalm, he declares who God says he is, what he believes God is to him, and what he believes God is doing in his life.

You can do the same thing. Start with any Scripture that is

meaningful and comforting to you and pray it out loud by making it into a personal declaration.

For example: "I am the Lord that heals you," becomes "You are the Lord that heals me" (Exodus 15:26). "No weapon turned against you will succeed," becomes "No weapon turned against me will succeed" (Isaiah 54:17). "I will satisfy them with a long life and give them my salvation," becomes "You will satisfy me with a long life and give me your salvation" (Psalm 91:16).

Or, in your prayer time, simply ask God what He wants you to know about yourself, about Him, and your circumstances. Wait and listen. Usually the first thing that comes to your mind is from God, so don't doubt. Declare out loud the truth He tells you. Let Him shower you with faithful promises and transform you into a new person that lives to honor and obey Him. His will for your life is pleasing and perfect, and there is no room for stinkin' thinkin.'

Father, thank you for the power of your word. Help me to declare your truth over myself in faith. Change my thinking, Lord! Amen.

30

REAL LIFE

Think about the things of heaven, not the things of earth. For you died to this life, and your real life is hidden with Christ in God
— Colossians 1:1-3

When we were young, we loved to play "make believe." We dressed up and pretended to be something we really weren't. Maybe it was a princess, a cowboy, or a rock star. It was fun to create a fantasy world where things were as we thought they should be. When play time ended, the costumes came off and we returned to "real life." We use these same words to describe a favorite actress in a movie. "In real life, she is married to so and so…" or "In real life, she has three children."

Real life may seem real — we can see, feel and touch the world around us. But Scripture is clear — what seems real today is temporal and will not last. Someday, "all of creation will be shaken and removed, so that only unshakable things will remain" (Hebrews 12: 27). Even people are like dust. Our earthly bodies are like wildflowers that bloom and die and blow away with the wind (Psalm 103:15-16). But our real life is not found in the visible world around us. Because of Christ, we are really temporary residents and foreigners here. Our true citizenship is in Heaven

(1 Peter 2:11; Philippians 3:20). Our real life is hidden in Christ in the unseen world. It's life as it should be.

Your real life is the life He created you to live. It is purposeful, satisfying, and overflows with Christ-like love and compassion. You are living in your "sweet spot," fulfilling your God-ordained destiny, and experiencing the abundant life Jesus promised you. To help us focus on our real life, Paul instructs us to think about things in Heaven. What is Heaven like? We know from Scripture that there are no human words to describe it: "No eye has seen, no ear has heard, and no mind has imagined what God has prepared for those who love him" (1 Corinthians 2:9). The Apostle John gives us a glimpse when He said that God will live among His people and He will wipe every tear from their eyes, and there will be no more death or sorrow or crying or pain (Revelation 21:3-4). There are also many people who have had near death experiences that confirm the various Scriptural accounts of Heaven. We know that Heaven is a place for rest, riches, and rewards. There will be eternal freedom from earthly pain and suffering, music, personal identity, fellowship, meaningful work, plants, animals, games, eating, drinking, rest, and security. Everything good and wonderful now will be better there.

When Paul instructs us not to think about things on earth, he doesn't mean we shouldn't engage in the world, but that we shouldn't be too attached to worldly things. We should look at our possessions, jobs, finances, talents, and even our physical bodies, through God's eyes, holding them loosely and knowing they are temporal. In a Scripture often read at funerals, Jesus promised He would prepare a place for us in His Father's home (John 4:2). That promise began the moment you invited Him to rule and reign in your life. In fact, at that very moment, your real life began. In that hidden place, you can have the peace that transcends all human understanding, the strength to face each day, and the power to be all He created you to be. In that place where your real life is hidden with Christ, you can be healthy, whole, satisfied, and complete. It sounds a lot like Heaven to me.

Father, thank you that my real life is hidden in Christ. Help me to see my life through the eyes of Heaven. Amen.

31

MAYHEM LIKE ME

Stay alert! Watch out for your great enemy, the Devil. He prowls around like a roaring lion, looking for someone to devour. Stand firm against him, and be strong in your faith. — 1 Peter 5:8-9

One of the best visual representations of your great enemy, the Devil, is the character "Mayhem" in the TV commercials. Webster defines mayhem as "needless or willful damage or violence." In the commercials, Mayhem personifies all the things that can wreck havoc on your possessions and threaten your life and safety. He becomes the satellite dish that falls off your roof and lands on your car, the raccoon that trashes your attic, and the team flag that flies off a car, covers your windshield and causes an accident. He's the jogger who distracts you and causes you to smash into a pole, the GPS that confuses you and causes your car to crash and the motorcycle shopper who takes your bike on a test drive and crashes it. When he's satisfied with the damage he's done, he walks away with a sinister laugh, warning us that we need a better insurance to protect us from "Mayhem like me." While these commercials make me laugh, they really do put a face on the Devil and show how he prowls around like a roaring lion looking for the next victim to devour.

In some of these commercials, Mayhem's victims are distracted, aren't paying attention, or have let their guard down. Others are simply innocent bystanders when Mayhem strikes, and totally unaware of the danger and damage that is about to be inflicted on them. Like Mayhem, the Devil's primary purpose is to steal, kill, and destroy the lives of innocent people (John 10:10). That's why Peter warns us to stay alert and strong in our faith and Paul admonishes us to be strong in the Lord's power so we can stand firm against the strategies and tricks of the Devil (Ephesians 6:11).

Lions attack sick, young and struggling animals, especially those who are weak, helpless, distracted, and alone. When we become so focused on our troubles that we forget to watch for danger, or we cut ourselves off from other believers, we are especially vulnerable to attack from the enemy. Be especially alert during these times. Keep your eyes focused on the truth of Scripture, just as Jesus did when He resisted Satan in the wilderness (Matthew 4:1-11). Be sure to call on the help of other Christians. Bring them into your battle and let them lift you up in prayer, especially when you're too weak to resist Mayhem on your own.

While you should always be alert, you don't have to worry about Mayhem lurking around to steal your health, plant his ugly lies, and ruin your day. Jesus already defeated him through His victory on the cross (Colossians 2:15). Then, He gave you authority over all the power of the enemy and promised nothing would injure you (Luke 10:19). You have the supernatural power of the Holy Spirit within you. You have access to the full body armor of God. Through His mighty power, you can resist the Devil's attacks, so that after the battle, you will still be standing firm (Ephesians 6:11-13). When you resist Mayhem with all your strategies and tricks, he has no choice but to flee from you (James 4:7). No more taunting and no more sinister laughing. You have the best insurance available to protect you from "Mayhem like me," and your policy is underwritten by Almighty God.

Father, thank you for giving me your supernatural power to stand firm against the enemy. Help me to stay alert and strong in faith so I can resist his strategies and tricks. Amen.

32

For Such a Time as This

But you have an anointing from the Holy One,
and you know all things. — 1 John 2:20

What is your anointing? What is your calling, your destiny, or your purpose in life? Every Christian has an anointing from God. It means that you were born for something special and have supernatural power from God to do exactly what He has called you to do. The word "anointing" actually means "to be smeared or rubbed with oil, especially for consecration." In the Scriptures, oil symbolizes the Holy Spirit. Whatever your calling, you have an anointing from the Holy One.

I never dreamed my anointing would be in pastoral ministry. Years before my diagnosis, I felt a distinct call to be a pastor and began exploring seminary, but chose not to pursue it. A strong calling began to rise up in me again after God healed me from cancer. For years, I wrestled with God. According to my husband, it was as if I was circling round and round the on ramp without ever getting on the freeway. Basically, I thought I could continue dabbling in the ministry of a pastor on my own terms without being fully surrendered to the call. I was afraid of what God would require of me, and I was afraid I wasn't ready.

Time passed and I kept circling the on ramp until one day, I heard a message by a well known pastor that resonated deeply with me. He said there are two parts to our identity; who we are on earth and how we are known in Heaven. After God reveals who we are in Heaven, He then has to deal with all our excuses for why we can't be who He called us to be. He said our destiny will not come to us. Once God reveals it, we need to step into it in faith. If we don't embrace who Heaven says we are, our resources dry up. But when we walk into our destiny, we walk in His provision. His message reminded me of Queen Esther. In her day, any woman who entered the king's courts while in session was killed, queen or no queen. But she knew she had to go in and expose Haman's evil plot to destroy Israel. Risking her life, she walked into the courts and delivered her message because she had a call to save a nation. She stepped out in faith, into her destiny, and God provided. She knew she was born for such a time as this (Esther 4:14).

I felt deeply convicted that night that I had been giving God my excuses and waiting for my destiny to come to me. As He expanded my ministry, I kept waiting to be ready for my calling. But God showed me that I will never be ready enough to be a pastor. Instead, I can decide to let Jesus make me ready and step out in faith. If I'm tempted to doubt my calling because I'm not worthy or unprepared, I can place myself in a position where His power will flow through me. Something supernatural happens to me when I minister to the sick and hurting. The Holy Spirit fills me with a Christ-like compassion that I don't carry in the natural. He especially likes to flow through the places in me where my human strengths can't get in the way. When I am weak, He is strong.

I finally got on the freeway. Following a rigorous review and interview process, my church commissioned me as a pastor. As I reflect on my calling, I've always felt like God pulled me out of the fire, covered me with supernatural armor, and threw me back in. There is a reason ten lepers were healed, but only one came back (Luke 17:11-19). In the natural, it's not easy to go back into the flames God rescued me from. I came back out of obedience, out of compassion, and out of gratefulness. I never want to forget what Jesus did for me.

What is your anointing? I don't know what you're called to do, but I know what the world needs. People need to know they have a righteous, holy, gracious and merciful Father who loves them. He is good, He is not the author of sin and disease, and He is not withholding His love or punishing them for falling short. They need to understand that they are precious in His sight and they can come as they are to the foot of the cross. His love for them is not a matter of what they do. They can never do enough to earn His love and there is nothing they have done that is beyond His Son's out-stretched arms of forgiveness. It's all about grace and what Jesus did for them. You might be the one God is calling to tell them. You might be born for such a time as this.

Father, thank you for the unique anointing you have placed on my life. Please give me the courage to step out in faith and into my destiny. Amen.

33

THE MYSTERY

Jesus replied, "If I want him to remain alive until I return, what is that to you? As for you, follow me." — John 21:22

Not too long ago I attended a beautiful celebration of life for a prominent woman of our church. There were over a thousand people there to share in the memories and celebrate all that she meant to her family, friends, and our congregation. She planned her own service and everything from the Scriptures and music, to the speakers and the food reflected her gifts and talents, her unique sense of humor, and her passion for life. She loved the Lord and she left a legacy behind that will impact the world for generations to come. She died after a long battle with advanced breast cancer, and had a special place in my heart. Thirteen years before, she received the exact same diagnosis as I would receive a year later. I followed her footsteps, but my path led to a much different place.

As survivors, we will always be troubled by stories like this one, especially when they hit so close to home. Our human minds start frantically searching for an explanation. Maybe some of us had better doctors or better treatments. Questions and comparisons about our past, our level of faith, our good deeds, and even devotion to the Lord can creep into our thinking. I warn you emphatically:

don't go there. God does not bring on sickness or disease to punish someone for their past, teach someone a lesson, or test their faith. Healing is not "God's will" for some and sickness is not someone else's "cross to bear." Faith is a gift from God, and we believers and the Church as a whole do not yet have a perfect faith. Jesus only chastised his disciples for their lack of faith, never the people who came to Him for healing. Nor, do our good deeds and our love for the Lord earn points with Him. He is no respecter of persons and He has no favorites. He died for all of us and all believers are equal in Christ (Acts 10:34; Romans 2:11).

So how do we reconcile the question? Why do some live and some die of the same diagnosis? One of my favorite quotes from Pastor Bill Johnson at Bethel Church in Redding, CA is that we must learn to walk in the revelation we have in the midst of the mysteries we can't explain. God is good and His Word is always true, regardless of what we see in the natural. We don't base theology on our experience. We base it on Jesus, our standard for all truth. We live in a constant tension between the supernatural realm and the natural. God heals whether we experience it or not. What we see around us must never shake our faith in what we know to be true. Shadrach, Meshach and Abednego capture this tension perfectly when they said: "If we are thrown into the blazing furnace, the God we serve is able to save us from it, and he will rescue us from your hand, O king. But even if he does not... " (Daniel 3:17-18). We must pray for the grace to praise God, regardless of the outcome, because we want Him more than we want healing.

After Jesus predicted Peter's death by crucifixion, Peter asked Him how John would die. Jesus told him it was none of his business and he shouldn't concern himself with it. Instead, He said:

"You follow me" (John 21:21-22). He didn't want us comparing ourselves with others to rationalize our own devotion to Him or to question God's judgment. Only God knows the heart of man. If we had Him all figured out and all our questions answered, there would be no need for faith. The mystery would be solved. Do you really want to worship a God who is no greater, no wiser, or no more powerful than you?

Father, thank you for the grace to praise you regardless of the outcome. Help me to walk in your revelation in the midst of the mysteries I can't explain. Amen.

34

DON'T DRINK THE POISON

I tell you, you can pray for anything, and if you believe that you've received it, it will be yours. But when you are praying, first forgive anyone you are holding a grudge against, so that your Father in heaven will forgive your sins, too. — Mark 11:24-25

As I was ministering to a woman with cancer recently, I learned of her difficult childhood. Her mother had abandoned the family when she was a little girl and her father passed away when she was a teenager. He was mostly disengaged and she grew up with no parental influence in her life. When I asked if she had forgiven them, she quickly responded, "Of course I have. I don't want to be like Jacob Marley dragging all those heavy chains around!" Even though she was un-churched until her illness, I was struck by her Biblical understanding of the consequences of unforgiveness. Somehow, she knew it would keep her bound up in chains like Scrooge's bitter business partner.

Jesus knew it too. He came to change all that. He came to release the captives and free the prisoners (Isaiah 61:1; Luke 4:18). There is a distinct difference between captives and prisoners. Captives are victims of someone else's sin. They are held in bondage against their will and did nothing wrong. But prisoners are held in bondage by their own choice. Often, they are locked up in the sin of unforgivenness. Jesus illustrates the consequences of unforgiveness in the story about the king who forgave a large debt owed by his servant. That same servant turned around and refused to forgive a smaller debt owed to him by a fellow servant. When the king heard this, he became angry and turned the servant over to jailers to be tortured until he paid back all he owed (Matthew 18:21-34). The next statement Jesus makes is one of the most difficult passages in the Bible to accept: "That's what my heavenly Father will do to you if you refuse to forgive your brothers and sisters from your heart" (Matthew 18:35).

Jesus commands forgiveness for our own good. He knows unforgiveness is a dangerous emotion that can hinder your prayers, block your blessing, destroy relationships, and lead to bitterness, hostility, physical illness, and mental stress. The symptoms of harboring resentment are hatred, a heavy heart, rehearsed arguments, vengeance, and avoidance. Some have said it's like drinking poison and expecting the other person to die. Most important, unforgiveness stands in the way of your intimacy with God. The choice is becoming clear. We can be miserable and drag around those heavy chains or we can forgive and be set free.

Forgiving someone who hurt you begins with understanding that you owe God a bigger debt than others owe you. Most of us have prayed the Lord's Prayer our entire life, but how many of us take it seriously when we ask God to "forgive us our sins, as we have forgiven those who sin against us" (Matthew 6:12)? I have often had to ask myself, do I really want this to be God's standard for forgiving me? Two verses later, Jesus drives the point home: "If you forgive those who sin against you, your heavenly Father will forgive you" (Matthew 6:14).

Right now, you might be thinking, "Do you have any idea what they did to me?" No, but Jesus does. He knows every hurt, every offense, and has cried every tear with you. He is no stranger to your pain. He knows forgiving them is nearly impossible to do on your own power. It's a choice you make, not a feeling or emotion. Once you make that choice, the Holy Spirit does the hard work, and eventually, your feelings will catch up. He can forgive when you can't. To choose to forgive someone doesn't mean what they did to you is okay or you are obligated to allow them access to hurt you again. It simply means that you have chosen to cancel the debt they owe you, give up the right to judge their motives, and give up your demand to get relief. Instead, you will let God heal your pain and provide the remedy.

To stay free, forgiveness has to become a lifestyle. You will have many opportunities today to be offended, whether it's a curt comment from a spouse or friend, someone who cuts you off on the freeway, or something much more serious. Please don't drink the poison. It's not good for your health.

Father, thank you for sending your Son to set me free. Please bring to my mind anyone I am holding a grudge against and help me to forgive them. Amen.

35

EXPECT GREAT THINGS

Listen to my voice in the morning, LORD. Each morning I bring my requests to you and wait expectantly. — Psalm 5:3

Are you confident when you pray that God hears you and will answer? Do you wait expectantly for the answers to come? God has been incredibly faithful to me in my prayer life and I have been blessed beyond anything I could ask or imagine. But, let me be honest. There have been times when I felt like my prayers were bouncing off the ceiling. There are some unanswered prayers deep in my heart that I've been waiting on for years. I'm sure there is movement forward in the spiritual realm, but from my vantage point, I see no movement at all. I can be tempted to give up and assume no answer means the answer is "no." But the Scripture says I must wait expectantly.

In this place of waiting, I'm reminded of a classic story written in 1828 by Emily Steele Elliot called *Expectation Corner*. It's about a man named Adam who lives in a redeemed land where a kind and loving king cared for his subjects. There were large storehouses on the land with everything they needed. All they had to do was make their requests and the king would send messengers out to deliver the supplies. The only condition was that they always needed to be found waiting and ready to receive the delivery when the king's messenger came. But Adam lived in poverty while all his neighbors lived in plenty. One day, a messenger took him to the storehouse and showed him all the packages of daily provision and gifts of favor addressed to his home. Sadly, he never received them because he never stood watch and answered the door. Adam finally comes to enjoy all the blessings of living in the land by learning how to petition and wait on the king for his daily needs.

We can be a lot like Adam. Maybe we don't request what we need because we feel unworthy. We think God won't provide for our needs because we have fallen short. This is certainly true; we all fall short. But that's why Jesus died. You are a redeemed child of God and there is no condemnation in Him (Romans 8:1). He has set you apart and is waiting to lavish His unlimited love and provision on you. Sometimes we lift up half-hearted prayers because we don't want to be disappointed if God doesn't answer. We don't want to get our hopes up, so in a sense, we give God an out. We pray without expecting to receive. When God comes with the answer, he finds the house dark and the door closed. Like Adam, we can't receive what we don't expect to receive. Sometimes, we just get tired of waiting. We stop asking altogether or we rush out ahead of God and take matters into our own hands. Instead of waiting for His best, we settle for much less and wonder why things aren't working out the way we had hoped.

Beloved child of God, you are a citizen of His Kingdom and entitled to all His blessings. You can rest assured that when you make a request, the King hears and the King will answer. Sometimes the answer might be different than you expect or it might take longer than you would like for your supply to come, but it will always be the King's very best. Bring Him your requests and expect great things. Stand watch at the door and be ready to receive. His storehouse is full of packages and promises addressed just to you.

Father, thank you that you hear my prayers and that you always answer. Help me to wait expectantly to receive all the blessings you have in store for me. Amen.

36

FULL MEAL DEAL

They were convinced by the power of miraculous signs and wonders and by the power of God's Spirit. In this way, I have fully presented the Good News of Christ from Jerusalem all the way to Illyricum. — Romans 15:18-19

When you order a sandwich at a fast food restaurant, you may be asked if you want to add a few items to complete the meal. While the Good News can't be compared to a quick lunch, it is certainly more than a one-course meal. The Good News of Christ is not only what Jesus said about salvation, but what He did. He didn't stop at preaching the message of eternal life. He healed the sick and cast out demons. When Peter preached to the Gentiles, he captured the essence of Jesus' ministry on earth: "God anointed Jesus of Nazareth with the Holy Spirit and with power. Then Jesus went around doing good and healing all who were oppressed by the Devil, for God was with Him" (Acts 10:37-38).

When Jesus was here, people had no problem accepting and believing that He could heal the sick. Their problem was in believing that He could forgive their sins and save their souls. Ironically, Christians today have no problem accepting Jesus as their "ticket to Heaven," but they struggle with believing He still heals the sick.

Then, as well as today, Jesus wants us to receive the *full* reward for His suffering. He wants you and me to live the abundant life of freedom He won for us on the cross. He wants to give us the "full meal deal."

To experience the fullness of salvation, we must first believe that physical healing, like the gift of eternal life, is part of the atonement given by grace through faith in Jesus Christ. Isaiah prophesied that He took our sicknesses and removed our diseases. He was beaten so we could be whole and we were healed by His stripes (Isaiah 53:4-5). Matthew acknowledged that when Jesus cast out evil spirits and healed all the sick, He fulfilled these words spoken through the prophet Isaiah (Matthew 8:16-17). Jesus Himself said, "For which is easier, to say, 'Your sins are forgiven you,' or to say, 'Arise and walk' " (Matthew 9:5)? Here He implied that forgiveness of sin and physical healing were both part of His redemptive grace. The ministry of Peter and Paul further exemplified that healing and miracles were a central and vital part of God's message to the world. When Peter prayed for boldness in preaching, He also asked the Lord for the power to do healing miracles through the name of Jesus (Acts 4:29-30). Paul was satisfied that he had *fully* presented the Good News by his message and by the miraculous signs and wonders he worked among the Gentiles (Romans 15:18-19).

The fullness of the Gospel is captured in the Greek word "sozo" used 110 times in the New Testament meaning "to save or make well or whole." The New Testament writers showed the completeness of the word by using it in different contexts to refer to three aspects of salvation. For example, in Romans 10:9, sozo means saved from eternal destruction: "That if you confess with your mouth Jesus is Lord and believe in your heart that God raised Him from the dead you shall be saved (sozo)." In Matthew 9:22, sozo refers to physical healing: "But Jesus turning and seeing her said, 'Daughter, take courage, your faith has made you well (sozo), and at once the woman was made well (sozo).' " And in Luke 8:36, sozo refers to inner healing or deliverance from demonic strongholds: "And those who had seen it reported to them how the man who was demon-possessed had been made well (sozo)."

Jesus died so you could receive the have rich, satisfying, abundant, and complete life. He wants you to receive your full reward for His suffering: salvation from eternal destruction, physical healing, and deliverance from demonic strongholds. He wants you to experience the full meal deal.

Father, thank you for the Good News of Christ Jesus! Help me to believe and receive by faith the fullness of my salvation: forgiveness for my spirit, healing for my body, and deliverance for my soul. Amen.

37

Diamond in the Rough

He will sit like a refiner of silver, burning away the dross. He will purify the Levites, refining them like gold and silver, so that they may once again offer acceptable sacrifices to the LORD. — Malachi 3:3

I'm not into bling. I'm not a really a "buy me a something that glitters for every special occasion" kind of girl. Actually, I'm more into jeans, boots, and leathers. It works well on the motorcycle. That's why I was shocked when my husband presented me with a tiny little box on our 35th wedding anniversary. Inside, was a beautiful, sparkling 1-carat diamond to replace a much smaller one on my engagement ring. I almost fell off my chair. My first thought was, "Who are you and what have you done with my husband?" Then I cried. It was truly a gift of love and affection. My new diamond sits proudly in its cathedral setting with cut out crosses on each side of the white gold band. I'm not into bling, but I love it.

Diamonds have a history of being everything from "a girl's best friend," to a symbol of love, wealth, or timeless beauty. The formation of my diamond began as far back as when the earth was formed, 100 to 250 miles deep within the earth's mantle, located between the center of the earth and thin layers of rocky crust near the surface. In that secret place, nature applied intense heat and pressure to carbon, transforming it into the hardest, most precious and lustrous gem in the entire world. Diamonds are a rare commodity, and only about 20 percent of them make their way up to the earth's surface and into a ring like mine.

As I admire my ring, it reminds me that we are a lot like diamonds. God will take His time with us as He transforms us into the precious gem He created us to be. Not unlike the intense pressure required to press carbon into crystalline form, the fiery trials of life press us into the mold that God envisioned before we were ever born (1 Peter 1:6-7). The refining fire of God continues to burn away the impurities of sin. Finally, seeing the hidden beauty within, the Master Jeweler transforms the rough stone into a beautiful faceted gem that shines and sparkles for the entire world to see.

The quality and value of diamonds are determined by a set of criteria that jewelers apply to their outward appearance. Diamonds with impurities and other inferior characteristics are downgraded in value. But God's diamonds are valued by something He sees on the inside — your character. Paul said we must not have "spot or wrinkle or any other blemish," but rather "be holy and without fault" (Ephesians 5:27). In His divine refining process, God uses the heat and pressure of everyday life to develop your endurance. Your endurance, in turn, will strengthen your character, deepen your trust in God, and give you unshakable hope in the future (Romans 5:3-5).

As you look toward your future and all God has in store for you, you are called to be the light of the world and to let your good deeds shine into the darkness for all to see (Matthew 5: 14-16). God raised you from the ashes of cancer and you are a powerful witness of His love and faithfulness. Through the cleansing blood of Jesus, He has refined you and transformed you from a diamond in the rough to a flawless gem. Let your life sparkle with the purity of a priceless diamond so people will see the beauty of Jesus shine through you. Even if bling is not their thing, they will find you irresistible.

Father, thank you for the transforming power of your divine refining process. Help me to shine the light of your Son into the dark places of the world. Amen

38

GOD WANTS YOU WELL

My people are destroyed for lack of knowledge. — Hosea 4:6

You can't receive what you don't know belongs to you. I have dental insurance, but if my employer never tells me that I have it, I'll continue to pay out of my own pocket as if I don't. If I'm not willing or able to carry the financial burden for my dental health on my own shoulders, I won't receive services at all. I'll leave the condition of my teeth up to fate. I'll never make a claim on what rightfully belongs to me.

A healthy body is God's plan for your life and a reflection of His goodness and His abundant love for you. If no one ever tells you that God wants you well, you will carry the burden of staying well on your own shoulders long after the cancer leaves your body. I've seen cancer survivors obsess over exercising, eating the right foods, and taking the right supplements. I've seen them log countless hours on the Internet keeping up to date on the latest research, and relentlessly pursue the best doctors and the latest medicines on the market. Staying well becomes an obsession that consumes as much of their lives as being sick. Please don't misunderstand. It's wise to take good care of our bodies and pay attention to our health habits, especially after dodging a bullet like cancer. It's important to partner with God to stay healthy, but let Him carry the burden. Remember, He alone is your Healer. You don't have to keep paying for His love and healing grace out of your own pocket.

If you don't know that God wants you well, and you have the mindset that the cancer came from Him, you may have found it difficult to ask Him to heal you. As a survivor, you may believe that staying well is also a matter of God's will. More than likely, you doctored during your cancer journey and you may be doctoring now for follow up care. Let me gently ask you this question: if it's not His will for you to be well, why did you seek medical help in the first place? If you believe it's possible for God to want you sick and you are seeking wellness through medical care, you would be acting against God's will. Instead of making a claim on what rightfully belongs to you, you are leaving your health up to fate or assuming whatever happens is God's plan.

The truth is, God planned for you to live a long and satisfying life (Psalm 91:16). He promised to be your God who would care for you throughout your lifetime — until your hair is white with age (Isaiah 46:4). Moses makes reference to God giving man a lifespan of seventy to eighty years (Psalm 90:10). Moses himself lived a long and full life of 120 years and died strong as ever and with clear eyesight (Deuteronomy 34:7). When the leper came to Jesus and said, "If you want to, you can make me well again," Jesus said with love and compassion, "I want to" and the man's leprosy disappeared (Mark 1:40-41). He wants to heal because it's His will to heal. It's His nature to heal. When we pray, "If it's your will, Lord, keep me well," we are really saying, "Lord, if it's not your will, then let this affliction take me." That doesn't sound like Jesus to me. Jesus healed everyone who came to Him. Nor does it align with the mandate He left with His disciples to "lay hands on the sick and heal them" (Mark 16:18).

The Word of God is like a priceless gift just waiting to be unwrapped. Inside you will find page upon page of blessing earmarked just for you. When you live in Him and His words live in you, God is ready to release all that he has in store for you (John 15:7). But you can't receive what you don't know belongs to you. Be careful not to miss out on His promises and all God wants you to know. He wants you well.

Father, thank you for the gift of a long and satisfying life. Help me to know your Word and receive all that belongs to me. Amen.

39

Pack Up and Leave

Resist the Devil and he will flee from you. — James 4:7

For a cancer survivor, the aches and pains of everyday life can take on a whole new meaning. Every new symptom can become the potential return of your disease. A simple headache or backache can unleash possibilities that can send you into an emotional tail spin. If your symptoms persist or fear itself lands you in the doctor's office, just the fact that you once had cancer can lead to tests they may never run otherwise, and even more anxiety as you wait for the results to prove you well. The Devil wants nothing more than to keep you in this cycle of fearing the worst. He wants to steal your healing and send you right back to where you started.

When Jesus walked on earth, one of His primary activities was to go around cleaning up the Devil's messes. God anointed Him with the Holy Spirit and with power so He could save, heal, and deliver the people Satan oppressed (Acts 10:38). Not surprisingly, Satan doesn't like it when God heals because it destroys his work. His primary objective is to steal, kill and destroy everything in his path (John 10:10).

One of the key strategies he uses to retaliate against Jesus is to steal His truth from us to try and bring back the former affliction.

Jesus warned us this could happen. In the parable of the sower, He said if we hear His Word and we don't understand it, Satan would come and snatch away what was sown in our heart (Matthew 13:19). Satan knows that God's Word brings healing and His Word is more powerful than sickness. He wants to destroy it before it gets firmly rooted in our heart. He knows if the Word is planted in good soil, a heart that understands and receives it, nothing will tempt us to fall away from the truth of our healing (Matthew 13:20-21). So he will try to bring on symptoms of sickness to convince us we really aren't healed. He wants to change our minds.

The enemy will persist in trying to get you to say yes and agree with your symptoms and believe his lies instead of God's promises. There will be plenty of opportunities to take his bait. This is not to say you shouldn't take heed of unusual physical symptoms and changes to your body. Your doctor will tell you what to watch for and what actions to take to best maintain your health after cancer. But you don't have to let the enemy use every ache and pain to control your life and steal the grace of healing that came directly from the hand of God.

You have a choice when the enemy threatens to take back what Jesus won for His glory. You can come in agreement with every physical symptom instead of God's promise of healing, and allow unbelief and fear attempt to re-establish sickness. You can live the rest of your life under dark clouds of doubt, never certain you are really healed, just waiting for the enemy to rise up and confirm your worst fear. Or, you can come in agreement with God and His Word and thank Him for all He has done. Tell the enemy that you are not going to believe his lies, no matter what. In the name of Jesus, tell him to pack up his symptoms and take them back to the enemy's camp. Resist him. He has no choice but to pack up and leave.

Father, thank you that your Word is firmly rooted in my heart. Help me to resist the lies of the enemy when he attempts to steal the truth of my healing. Amen.

40

TELL THE WORLD

Tell the nations what he has done. Let them know how mighty he is! Sing to the LORD, for he has done wonderful things. Make known his praise around the world. — Isaiah 12:4-5

I love getting emails from readers. It blesses me to know that some teaching or revelation God has inspired me to write has impacted the life of another child of God. I received such an email recently from a cancer survivor who expressed her gratefulness for a book I had written that got her back into the Bible and gave her the comfort she so desperately needed. Praise God! Then she asked for prayer and wisdom. Her pastor had asked her to share her story with the entire congregation. She didn't consider herself a good public speaker, but she couldn't keep the news about God's love and faithfulness hidden from those around her. Even though she was nervous about speaking in public, she had no choice but to tell the world how Jesus had changed her life.

It's natural for us to share the name of a good hairdresser or a skillful doctor, recommend a good book or movie, or let our friends in on the good news when we discover a great bargain or a new boutique. But for some reason, we hesitate to tell them the greatest news of all. David didn't hesitate. He waited patiently for the Lord to hear his cries for help, and the Lord heard. He saved David by rescuing him from the pit of despair and placing him securely on solid ground. Then, He guided each step as David walked steadily forward in faith giving thanks for all God had done (Psalm 40:1-2). David couldn't resist telling the world about God's unfailing love and faithfulness. He was not afraid to speak out. He simply couldn't keep such good news hidden in his heart (Psalm 40:9-10). The people who saw the new song of praise on David's lips were so astounded by what the Lord had done in His life that they too put their trust in the Lord (Psalm 40:3).

You may never be called to preach to your congregation. You may never be called to write books, become a pastor, or a great Bible teacher. But God has called you to declare His good works to those around you (Psalm 73:28). When He lifted you out of the pit of cancer, the people in your life were watching. Now, they want to know how you're doing. They want to know if you are sick or well and how you survived the ordeal. Sometimes they don't have the courage to ask, but often they do. Each time a person asks, you have the opportunity to testify to His faithfulness and saving power. You have the opportunity to tell them how He heard your cries, lifted you out of the pit of despair, and set your feet on solid ground. As you praise Him with a new song on your lips, many will see what he has done in your life and be amazed. They will put their trust in the Lord simply because you made a decision to tell the world.

Father, thank you for rescuing me from the pit of cancer and setting my feet on solid ground. Help me to sing your praises and tell the world of your unfailing love and faithfulness at every opportunity. Amen.

41

GOD OR GOOGLE?

When the Spirit of truth comes, he will guide you into all truth. He will not speak on his own but will tell you what he has heard. He will tell you about the future. He will bring me glory by telling you whatever he receives from me. — John 16:13-14

If I need a recipe for artichoke dip or chili, I Google it. If I'm looking for vacation rental homes in Disney World, I Google it. It's not a problem if I have some ache or pain and I want to save a trip to the doctor; I just Google my symptoms. In fact, I can Google and find information on just about every personal problem imaginable, whether it's related to health, finances, relationships, or work. Occasionally, I've found myself struggling with some really perplexing question, just wishing Google could give me an answer. If I'm not careful, I can be tempted to rely on the voices of the world instead of the voice of God. Instead of consulting my personal Counselor, Google will dictate my thoughts, words, and actions.

Before Jesus died, He promised His followers He would send a Counselor, the Holy Spirit, to remind them of His truth, what He did, and what He said. The Spirit of God would convince the world of its sin and call for repentance. He would reveal God's standard of right living for all believers because Jesus would no longer be physically present on earth (John 16:8-10). The Counselor would live in all who believe and would never leave us (John 14:16-17). He would also help us discern right from wrong, and teach us how to live according to God's plan for our lives, both here and now and in the future.

What a privilege to know that Father God speaks directly to the Holy Spirit living within us! Through our personal Counselor, we have direct access to God's plan for our lives. We can be tempted to allow the voices of the world to drown out His voice. The Apostle Paul advises us to live according to our new life in Christ, so we won't do what our sinful nature craves (Galatians 5:16). When the Holy Spirit guides and controls us, the Word of Christ will be in our minds, His love will guide our actions and His power will help us live according to His purposes, not the world.

It's a daily choice to center our lives on God. We can seek the world's counsel in every perplexing situation, or we can ask what Jesus wants us to do and let the Holy Spirit point us in the right direction. Paul further warns that the way of the world leads to death, but His way brings life and peace (Romans 8:5-6). Living in the Spirit instead of the flesh allows us to hear God's voice, receive His protection, grow in Christ, and become all that He has called us to be.

Google isn't a bad thing. It brings knowledge to our fingertips. We can find instant answers to virtually everything. Solomon, the wisest man to ever live, reminds us that there is a difference between having knowledge and applying that knowledge to everyday life. Application of knowledge is wisdom, and true wisdom comes directly from the heart of God. He warns us not to depend on our own knowledge or be impressed with our own wisdom, but to seek God's will and let Him direct our paths (Proverbs 3:5-7). God gave you a personal Counselor, the Holy Spirit, to do just that. He will guide you into all truth and tell you all that He has heard from the Father about your future. You can go through life consulting the voices of the world, or you can fall on your knees and seek His perfect plan. God or Google? You decide.

Father, thank you for the gift of your Holy Spirit. Help me discern your voice of truth and wisdom above all the competing voices of the world. Amen.

42

Idols of the Heart

*Dear children, keep away from anything that might take
God's place in your hearts.* — 1 John 5:21

I don't just love my phone, I *love* my phone. I have been told I
need a 12-step program for smart phone junkies. I love having four
email accounts, Internet news, my calendar, text messaging, music,
camera, and hundreds of apps all at my fingertips. I've been known
to have an anxiety attack if I'm traveling out of service range or if
the battery is low and there is no possibility of re-charging. I have
to be very conscious about keeping my phone put away during
conversations with people, and not letting it distract me during the
time I set aside for prayer and fellowship with God. My phone can
easily become an idol.

An idol is any thing, activity, or idea that we place higher than
God. There are the obvious things that come to mind when we
think about worshipping idols. Most of us know that bowing
down to a golden calf or Buddha statue is wrong. When I traveled
to Sri Lanka and India, there were Jesus statues everywhere. He
had become an idol right along with Buddha and their 330 million
Hindu gods. Even good things can become idols. Sometimes we
idolize food, sports, money, computers, TV shows, work, our

spouse, our children, our church activities, and yes, our smart phones. Our blessings can become idols when we value them more than God. It happens when our trust moves subtly from the Creator to His creation. We don't realize how much trust we have placed in our possessions, health, relationships, or our personal strengths until they are suddenly threatened or stripped away. As a cancer survivor, you know what it feels like to trust in your body and then face the real possibility of losing your health.

When we don't fully understand God's place in our lives, we will worship something else. Whether it happens unknowingly or out of rebellion, it breaks God's heart and causes a wall between us. We can know in our head that replacing God with something else is like replacing the sun with a 30-watt light bulb, but we can be tricked into making bad choices. One of Satan's tricks is to distract us from pure and sincere worship of Christ (2 Corinthians 11:3). Satan even tempted Jesus. When he offered Jesus all the kingdoms of the world if He would kneel down and worship him, Jesus rebuked him and quoted the Scriptures: "You must worship the Lord your God; serve only him" (Matthew 4:8-10). Jesus shows us how to respond when Satan tempts us to worship idols.

If we don't resist, God's response is jealousy (Exodus 20:5). The Israelites got tired of waiting for Moses to come down from the mountain with God's covenant, so they made a golden calf to worship and indulged in pagan rivalry. Moses pleaded with God and he withdrew His threats to destroy the entire nation, but there were consequences for their idol worship (Exodus 32:1-14). Even though we live under grace on the other side of the cross, God is still jealous for the affections of our hearts and feels betrayed when we place other things higher than him.

Worshipping idols will never satisfy the deep longing in your soul that only God's presence will satisfy. Your satisfaction will always be superficial and short-lived. Idols simply cannot give deep inner peace your soul craves. That's why the Apostle John wrote these powerful words: "Do not love this world nor the things it offers you, for when you love the world, you do not have the love of the Father in you. For the world offers only a craving for physical pleasure, a craving for everything we see, and pride in our achievements and possessions. These are not from the Father, but are from this world. And this world is fading away, along with everything that people crave. But anyone who does what pleases God will live forever" (1 John 2:15-17).

What is taking God's place in your heart today? It may be time to repent and renounce any idols that have snared your soul. Worship Him with all your heart in all you think, say, and do and be truly filled with His pleasure and joy!

Father, please point out anything in my life that I have placed higher than you. Forgive me for the times I've worshipped at any alter other than yours. Amen.

43

You Want Me to Do What?

Mary responded, "I am the Lord's servant, and I am
willing to accept whatever he wants. May everything you have
said come true." — Luke 1:38

Shortly after completing cancer treatment and receiving my healing, I attended a Susan G. Komen Race for the Cure®. As I looked over a sea of pink — 47,000 men, women, and children, all touched in some way by breast cancer — a silent voice spoke from deep within me: "I don't want you to race for them. I want you to pray for them." My first reaction was, "God, is that really you?" After I realized I really did hear the voice of God speak gently to my spirit, my second reaction was, "You want me to do what!?" I knew nothing about praying for people. I had never prayed out loud before for anyone in my life. I didn't know how to minister to the sick. But somehow I knew this was part of my destiny.

Sometimes I wonder if I felt a little bit like another Mary when God asked her to do the impossible. She knew being pregnant out of wedlock in her culture spelled disaster unless the father of the child agreed to marry her. If her own father rejected her, she would be forced into begging or prostitution. If she told the truth about what God asked her to do, she would be called crazy as well. But

Mary responded willingly in spite of all the risks and unknowns. She only knew that God was asking her to serve Him.

My call is nothing like Mary's, but with God's help, I mustered up enough courage after race day to found Pray for the Cure, a church-based healing prayer and discipleship ministry for people struggling with all types of cancer. Since 2001, people have come to share their hopes and fears with others facing cancer, listen to encouraging stories from survivors, receive Bible teaching, and experience healing prayer and anointing in a confidential setting. As a leader and pastor of Pray for the Cure, I have been privileged to pray for, encourage and disciple countless people with all types of cancer in the prayer chapel, in hospitals, hospices, and by phone and email. God has healed many of them. None of this would have been possible without His grace.

God has a special calling on your life, too. One way or another, He will use the cancer the enemy intended for evil to bring Himself glory. I encourage you not to limit yourself to things you can do for God on your own power. Instead, listen for the things He has called you do to that you cannot do without His grace and the power of the Holy Spirit. You may have to let Him put you in a place of discomfort like that first time I prayed for someone with cancer. I promise He will use these impossible tasks to mold and stretch you into the person He has called you to be. And may your response always be, "I am the Lord's servant."

Father, thank you for causing everything to work together for good. Give me the courage and power to answer your call on my life, in spite of all the risks and unknown outcomes. Amen.

44

One Thing

The one thing I ask of the LORD — the thing I seek most — is to live in the house of the LORD all the days of my life, delighting in the LORD's perfections and meditating in his Temple. — Psalm 27:4

Sometimes when I read this passage in Scripture, I think of Curly in the movie *City Slickers* (©1991 Metro-Goldwyn-Mayer Studios Inc.). The plot is about a New Yorker named Mitch who is suffering from a mid-life crisis. His two friends, in crises of their own, present him with a birthday gift: a two-week Southwestern cattle drive for the three of them. The movie is all about the antics and adventures of these three city slickers as they learn the ropes and move the herd to Colorado.

This is not a particularly life changing movie that will have great Kingdom impact, but there was one scene in the middle of the long drive where tough-as-nails trail boss Curly gives Mitch some life advice. "Do you know what the secret of life is?" he asks Mitch. Holding up one finger, he answers his own question: "This." Confused and a bit sarcastically, Mitch asks, "Your finger?" Curly answers, "One thing. Just one thing." Then he tells him if he would just stick to that one thing, the rest wouldn't matter. Of course Mitch wants to know what the one thing is, and Curly answers, "That's what you have to find out."

What's your one thing? David discovered his: "To live in the house of the Lord all the days of my life, delighting in the Lord's perfections and meditating in his Temple." David may be referring to the special tent that he had prepared for the Ark of the Covenant (2 Samuel 6:17). Or he may have been referring to the Tabernacle of Moses that was filled with the awesome glory of the Lord during the Israelites journey out of captivity. When the cloud of the Lord that rested on the Tabernacle lifted and moved, they would set out on their journey and follow it (Exodus 40:34-37). Some 500 years later, David's son Solomon built the Temple, replacing the Tabernacle as the central place of worship. In either case, the Temple represented the "presence of God." David's greatest desire was to live in His presence and worship Him, all the days of his life. Based on Curly's theology, this was the one thing in David's life that really mattered.

The Temple was God's home on earth, filled with the overwhelming sense of His presence. We don't have to go to a church or a building to experience the His presence. After Jesus died and rose from the dead, God no longer needed a physical building to dwell on the earth. His Temple is now His Church, the body of believers, and His Spirit inhabits each one of us.

Just as David took joy in experiencing God's presence in the Temple, you can delight in the perfection of His presence within you. He is the perfect Shepherd who will guide you, protect you, and lead you in the way you should go. He can heal all your hurts and fill all the voids that cancer stole from you. Surrender all your goals for your health, family, work, friends, finances, and hobbies to the One Thing, the One Sovereign God who reigns over all of it. His plans for you are perfect and He knows the desires of your heart even better than you. Follow Curly's advice. Stick to that One Thing, and the rest won't matter at all.

Father, thank you for the gift of your presence. Help me to seek you with all my heart until nothing else matters. Amen.

45

SHOW ME YOUR GLORY

Moses responded, "Then show me your glorious presence."
— Exodus 33:18

Moses knew his assignment. God directed him to take the Israelites to the Promised Land. But after the golden calf fiasco, God told Moses He wouldn't travel with them because they were a stubborn, unruly people. Moses continued to spend time with God in the Tent of Meeting, until one day he asked the Lord who He would send with him so he could complete his assignment. He reminded God that the Israelites were His very own people and asked for more of the favor God had shown toward him in the past. God assured Moses that He would personally travel with him and everything would be fine. Pushing further, Moses pleaded with the Lord not make them go without His presence. God again assured Moses that He would do what he asked, but Moses continued to push. He asked God to prove it. He wanted to see the manifest presence of God as assurance of God's presence with him (Exodus 33:1-18). So God revealed Himself to Moses in a pillar of cloud and passed in front of him (Exodus 34:5-6).

We all have God assignments. He has a unique plan and purpose for each of us. As a survivor, in addition to your family, work, and other activities, you will have many opportunities to join in the cause of fighting cancer, finding a cure, or caring for the sick and suffering. Whether you plan and organize or simply participate, there may be races, relays, walks, rides, support groups, prayer meetings, products to buy or sell, books to write, ministries to start, and speeches to give. All of these are good things to do, and some might be direct assignments from God. But not all of them are your assignment. Moses prayed for God's presence to be with him before he moved forward. God told Moses that He would personally go with him and give him rest (Exodus 33:14). When we do good things for God without His presence and favor, we don't experience rest. We experience burnout.

How do you know an assignment is from God? How do you know God's presence is with you? God is omnipresent and His presence is everywhere, at all times. David said there was no place we could go to hide from Him (Psalm 139:7). His presence in the form of the Holy Spirit also dwells within each believer (1 Corinthians 13:16). If the presence of God is always around us and in us, what we are really hungering for is the realization of His presence and our ability to perceive it. We encounter His presence when we become fully conscious of His love, mercy, grace, compassion, peace, comfort, and rest.

If God is a part of what you are doing, you will know it. His Spirit will speak to yours. He will show you favor. You will experience His peace, even if the assignments He has given you are difficult. If you move forward without Him, you may receive a check in your spirit. You may feel as though you are pushing a boulder up hill. You will not experience His rest and your schedule may feel as if it's out of control. Not every assignment from God will be quick and easy, but there is always time for rest. There is always enough time to do what He calls you to do. If you have any doubt an assignment is from God, stop and pray the prayer of Moses. Lord, if this is from you, show me your glory!

Father, thank you for the plans and purposes you have for my life. Please help me discern my Kingdom assignments. Show me your glorious presence! Amen.

46

THE SEASONS OF LIFE

*I have called you back from the ends of the earth, saying,
'You are my servant.' For I have chosen you and will not throw
you away.* — Isaiah 41:9

I never aspired to serve on the elder board of a 6000 member
mega church. I certainly never aspired to be president. When we
follow a path of obedience, we have no idea where God might
lead. Often, it's not on a path of our own choosing. After my year
long journey through cancer, God led me to a place of high level
leadership and service in my local congregation. I would never have
taken this path if it were left up to me. The mantle of responsibility
was not something I was willing or able to carry on my own power,
not to mention the time commitment. Eventually, I grew to really
enjoy how God was using my gifts to advance His Kingdom. I was
a living testimony of His promise to take what the enemy intended
for evil and causing it to work together for good (Romans 8:28).
I was honored to serve in this role for ten satisfying and fruitful
years. And then it ended as abruptly as it began.

Change is a normal part of life. Perhaps you find yourself in
a season of change right now. Maybe your children have all left
home and you're adjusting to an empty nest. Or maybe you're

facing job loss or retirement or relocating to another city. Perhaps, like me, you are closing the chapter on something that gave you great satisfaction after God triumphed over the cancer that tried to destroy your life. Whatever has thrust you into a season of change, you might feel as though you've been pulled up by the roots. God was using all your gifts for His glory. You were in your sweet spot and everything made sense. And now it doesn't. If you're totally honest, you might admit to feeling tossed aside, wondering what God will do next, or worse, if He's finished with you.

Just as the seasons in nature, there are seasons in our journey of faith (Ecclesiastics 3:1). God orchestrates these seasons to maximize our spiritual growth as well as the spiritual fruit we produce for His Kingdom. We need to recognize the season we are currently in and be able to live, minister, and serve accordingly. If we compare these seasons to the seasons of nature, spring is a time of new adventures and new opportunities. Perhaps God is birthing a new ministry, a new relationship, or new revelation about His nature and His ways. Summer is a time to bear fruit and grow spiritually. You may sense God's presence and anointing more powerfully and be blessed by a growing, active ministry. You may be in your sweet spot. Autumn often takes you to a place of downsizing, either in practical areas such as time and finances, or your ministry and volunteer commitments. You may feel compelled to return to the disciplines of spending time with the Lord through prayer, worship, and His Word.

Finally, winter is a season of spiritual rest. It is not a time for bearing fruit. It is a time of waiting silently before God. Sometimes we get tired of waiting for the "next thing" so we try to make something happen. We commit to things we shouldn't in order to feel productive. Winter can feel cold and bleak, as if God is not hearing our prayers or speaking to us. Sometimes we might feel confused and wonder: "God rescued me from the pit of cancer, called me back from the ends of the earth to serve Him, only to throw me away?"

If you find yourself in a winter season, or even a season of pulling back and preparing for the winter to come, stay focused on God. Reflect on His goodness, His faithfulness, and His promises. Maintain and attitude of reverence before Him. Remember, God rested too. Most of all, remember that spring always comes. During this time of Sabbath rest, He is preparing you for a season of new adventures, new assignments, and new opportunities. He created you so you could do the good things He planned for you long ago (Ephesians 2:10). Heaven is counting on you. He will not throw you away.

Father, thank you for orchestrating the seasons of life to cause me to grow and bear fruit for your Kingdom. Help me to stay connected to you even when I'm confused and don't know your plan. Amen.

47

IN THE PINK

The thief's purpose is to steal and kill and destroy. — John 10:10

Almost everyone knows the significance of pink ribbons. It all started in 1992 when Evelyn Lauder and her husband, an executive for the Estee Lauder cosmetics company, largely financed the distribution of little bows given to women at department store makeup counters to remind them about breast cancer. That effort grew into pink fundraising products, everything from pink Bibles to pink kitchen appliances, congressional designation of October as Breast Cancer Awareness Month, and millions of dollars in donations to breast cancer care and research. Susan G. Komen for the Cure® was formed ten years earlier and has grown into the largest source of nonprofit funds dedicated to the fight against breast cancer in the world, having invested more than $1.9 billion to the cause of saving lives and finding cures. The campaign against breast cancer has expanded to nearly every facet of society. Even professional sports teams and players have collaborated with various fund raising initiatives and shown their support through pink shoes, pink cleats, pink caps, pink jerseys, helmet decals, pink balls, pink gloves, and pink wristbands.

I am profoundly grateful to the pioneers of this movement and to everyone who has organized or participated in any event dedicated to creating awareness and raising money for the fight against breast cancer. These efforts have been extremely important to the lives of all women. As a survivor, I've participated in these events myself many times. But, I have to admit I have mixed emotions when I see pink in virtually every place I shop, and everywhere I look. Sometimes the commercialism bothers me. Every business has figured out how to jump on the pink bandwagon and make a profit off of breast cancer by sharing a small portion of their profit with the good cause of fighting it. I'd feel better buying a pink toaster or a furnace cleaning and knowing that 100 percent of the profit went to the cause. I actually find the color pink to be a bit unsettling. It reminds me of "in the pink," a phrase that originally referred to "in the best possible health." The bottom line is that breast cancer is not a "pink experience." In fact, without the Lord carrying me through it, it would have been very much the opposite!

There's a part of me that wonders if all this pink gives a little more glory to Satan than he deserves. Satan, the author of sickness and disease, is the mastermind behind breast cancer. I wonder if he sits back embracing all the pink and takes pride in the pain and suffering He has caused the women in this world. He attacks them at the very core of their femininity. His goal is to steal from them, kill them, and destroy them. This was never God's plan for His beloved daughters. In the Garden of Eden, man and woman were created to live forever in paradise with no sickness or disease. But God loved us so much that He gave us free choice to follow Him. Unfortunately, Adam and Eve chose poorly. Sin came into the world with the fall, and along with it, cancer. But Jesus came to restore what Satan stole and give us a life of abundance. He died and conquered death and disease once and for all (Isaiah 53:4-5). He gave us the Holy Spirit as a down payment on our future glory (Romans 8:19-23)!

We can run our races and buy pink products, but let's make sure to focus our hearts on the healing work of Jesus, and not on the destructive work of the enemy. Instead of telling the world how big our problem is, let's tell the world how big our Jesus is. We will never find a complete solution exclusively through human efforts. We will never find a complete solution apart from Christ. In Him, we are truly in the pink.

Father, thank you for the efforts of countless people who have fought the earthly battle against cancer. Help me to proclaim and celebrate your final victory over Satan and his destructive work. Amen.

48

GREEN PASTURES

*The LORD is my shepherd; I shall not want. He makes me
to lie down in green pastures; He leads me beside the still waters.
He restores my soul.* — Psalm 23:1-3 (NKJV)

Are you looking for direction in your life? Are you searching for an answer to a troubling problem? Are you hurting inside? Are you struggling with relationship difficulties? Are you feeling the burden of responsibilities and commitments? Are you struggling to break free of a particular sin in your life? Are you feeling compelled to try something new and need the Lord's strength to move forward? Are you feeling spiritually dry and longing to re-connect with God? Are you simply longing for more intimacy with God? If you answered "yes" to any of these questions, soaking is for you!

My first encounter with soaking was in India after a particular grueling day of ministry. The poverty in the surrounding slums was unfathomable and the needs of the people overwhelming. The team felt dry and spent. Our leaders knew we could not continue ministering from a place of emptiness. We had poured out our hearts on the people and had nothing left to give. We couldn't give away what we didn't have. So they cancelled the ministry time scheduled for the next morning and introduced us to soaking.

"Soaking" is another term for "waiting on the Lord" or to "tarry." Soaking satisfies a deep longing for God that He hardwired into every human heart. In each of us, He created a deep God-sized hole that only He can fill. It was all part of His plan to live in fellowship with us. As believers, we have the promise of the Holy Spirit living inside us. But living in this world with all the stresses and strains and pouring out His love to those around us causes us to leak! Soaking is a way to stop, rest, and refill. It is a time we set aside to be with Father God with no shopping lists and no agendas. It is not a time of striving prayer, but a time to rest in His presence and be still in His arms of love.

Soaking begins by finding a quiet place to rest. You can lie down or sit in a chair, whatever is most comfortable. Soft intimate worship music will help you quiet your soul and prepare you to draw close to Father God. Start by quieting your thoughts and focusing your mind on Jesus. As you wait for your thoughts to settle, invite the Holy Spirit to come. Surrender your mind, soul, and body to Him. Open yourself to receive and give the Holy Spirit permission to reveal Himself according to His will. Focus on His presence and don't try to analyze things. Just rest in faith and trust that God's presence is working within you. It might take awhile for your mind to clear and for you to come to a place of rest. Try to allow at least 15 minutes. The more you soak, the more time you will want to spend in His presence.

Since coming home from India, I have made soaking a habit and have a large collection of soaking music. My favorite time and place to soak is in my bed at night with my iPod. As you begin soaking in God's presence, you will discover what I discovered — you will emerge from your time of rest feeling refreshed and lighter, as though the weight of the world has been lifted. This should come to no surprise. Jesus beckoned the tired and heavy laden to come to Him for rest. In His gentle, humble presence, He promised to lift your burdens (Matthew 11:28-30). Start soaking today and let Him restore your soul. Let Him lift your burdens, renew your love for Him, and fill you with His Spirit. As a soaker, you can't help but impact the world around you because you carry His presence wherever you go. You find it easier to love others, even difficult people, because your love tank is full. You are a kinder, gentler, more patient you — all because you make a habit of lying down in green pastures.

Father, thank you for the gift of your presence. Help me make a habit of lying down in green pastures and letting you restore my soul. Amen.

49

THROUGH HEAVEN'S EYES

But to all who believed him and accepted him,
he gave the right to become children of God. They are reborn —
not with a physical birth resulting from human passion or plan,
but a birth that comes from God. — John 1:12-13

People of all genders, ages, and backgrounds come to Pray for the Cure, our monthly healing and discipling ministry for people touched by cancer. Sometimes people facing a diagnosis will bring a close friend or family member along for support. Sometimes they come alone. They may come from our congregation, other churches, or no church at all. Some come from other cities and even other states. Each one has a unique story. Some have been recently diagnosed, and others are in the midst of treatment. Some are survivors who share their testimony of healing to give others hope.

A few years ago, a woman came to the group adorned in pink ribbon accessories. I assumed she was going through treatment or recently diagnosed with breast cancer, until I learned she was long time survivor of early stage disease. She was checking out Pray for the Cure after being a part of another support group for the past 12 years. Another time, a frightened young woman came who didn't have cancer, but she had cancer in her family and wanted to be prepared. She wept and wanted support for the cancer she just knew would come someday.

What is your story? Whatever it may be, Heaven doesn't see a cancer patient, a future cancer patient, or even a cancer survivor. Heaven sees a child of God, a new creation, reconciled to God by faith, and redeemed, forgiven, and healed by the blood of Jesus (Romans 5:1; Colossians 1:13-14). He loved you first, called you out of darkness and into the light, and adopted you into very own His family (1 Peter 2:9; 1 Thessalonians 4:1). Just as an adopted child gains all rights of a legitimate child in his new family, you are a full heir to His estate. You have all the privileges and responsibilities of a child in His family and access to all His blessings, treasures, and gifts (Romans 8:14-15; Ephesians 1:3-8). You may know all your flaws and remember your mistakes, but Heaven sees you as righteous and holy (Ephesians 4:24). You may remember the cancer that was part of your life, but Heaven has forgotten it.

As a child of a King, your royal position is secure. There is no condemnation in Him (Romans 8:1). There is no good thing you can do that will make you love Him more and no mistake you could ever make that would cause Him to love you less (Romans 8:35-39). He will work for good through all your mistakes, the mistakes of others against you, and love you through any trial or difficulty you will ever face (Romans 8:28). Through Christ, you don't live under the shadow of cancer. You live in victory as a citizen of Heaven where no evil can touch you (Philippians 3:20; 1 John 5:18).

Your status as a citizen of Heaven comes with the privileges of royalty. As a brother or sister of King Jesus, you are seated with Him in the heavenly realm (Ephesians 2:6). Everything that belongs to Jesus belongs to you, including the right to go boldly before Daddy's throne with freedom and confidence (Ephesians 3:13; Romans 8:17). You have unique gifts and a special calling on your life, and have been chosen and appointed to bear fruit for His Kingdom (John 15:16; 1 Corinthians 12:27).

Knowing your true identify in Christ makes all the difference in how you approach your life. Will you choose to walk everyday in the freedom Jesus died for? Will you live the life your Father in Heaven created you to live, or will you live the life the enemy wants to steal from you? Your Father never intended for His children to live with cancer, or the possibility of cancer, or the fear of cancer coming back. Through Heaven's eyes, you are a son or daughter of Almighty God resting safely and securely in His loving arms, with a destiny and purpose to fulfill for His glory. Through Heaven's eyes, you are the child you were born to be.

Father, thank you for loving me, for choosing me as your very own possession, and adopting me into your family. Please help me to see and live every day of my life through the eyes of Heaven. Amen.

50

GRANDMA ROAD

But joyful are those who have the God of Israel as their helper,
whose hope is in the LORD their God. He made heaven and earth,
the sea, and everything in them. He keeps every promise forever.
— Psalm 146:5-6

His name is Phillip Xavier Nelson and he loves anything with
wheels — especially trucks. "Xsie," as we call him, knows every
truck by name. Some of his favorites are dump trucks, garbage
trucks, crane trucks, cement mixers, 18-wheel semi trucks, tow
trucks, flatbed trucks, and fire trucks. He can even say ex-ca-va-tor.
That's quite a mouthful for a two year old. You can imagine the
excitement of riding in the car for a little guy who loves trucks,
cars, motorcycles, and trains. I have a whole new appreciation for
the diversity of equipment on a typical construction site. Eighteen
wheelers are his latest obsession. He steers, shifts, and honks the horn
while he "drives" his car seat down the busy freeway passing all the
other semi trucks. Basically, Xsie views the world as something to
drive on. He will make a road out of anything, anywhere, anytime,
including Grandma. I like being "Grandma Road" so he can drive
his Mac truck up and down my leg that forms a bridge from the
coffee table to the couch! This Grandma is convinced of one thing;

Xsie is the cutest, sweetest, most adorable little boy on the planet, bar none.

Everyone told me that being a grandma was the best thing ever, but for me, the joy of spending time with Xsie is a double blessing. Twelve years ago, while bald, broken, and going through cancer treatment, I didn't always allow myself to dream about my future. For a while, I wasn't sure I would ever meet my grandchildren. But God is faithful and His faithfulness extends to every generation (Psalm 119:90). We can trust him, rely on him, and depend on him totally and without reservation. Shortly after my treatment ended, I began to stand on this basic truth about our Father in Heaven. I needed to believe the certainty of God, or I would forever live under a dark cloud of uncertainty and allow myself to be tossed and turned by the winds of change.

In a world that is uncertain and constantly changing, God is constant and does not change (Malachi 3:6). The character of God is reflected in Jesus and He is the same yesterday, today, and forever (Hebrews 13:8). His love never fails, never changes, and lasts forever (Psalm 100:5). The grass and flowers may wither away, but His Word is eternal, unfailing, and constant (Isaiah 40:8). God is our solid rock. We can stand on Him and know He never moves, regardless of the shifting world around us.

If God doesn't change, then we can trust Him to do what says He will do. We can trust Him to always keep His promises (Numbers 23:19). He stands by the commitment He made to a thousand generations (Psalm 105:8). No matter what difficulties we encounter, whether in the past, present, or future, we can count on His blessings. He heals us, ransoms us from death, surrounds us with His tender mercies, and fills our life with good things (Psalm 103:3-5).

God fulfilled another promise today. Another good thing has come into my life. After a precarious pregnancy for both mother and child — after nine months of bathing her in prayer — Nadia Lilanna Nelson came into the world. Given the conditions surrounding her mother's pregnancy, the doctor called little "Lila" a miracle. And she is…a beautiful, healthy, precious miracle from Heaven. I think back to where I was twelve years ago and my heart overflows with joy. My God who made the heavens and earth, my helper and my only hope, keeps every promise forever! Another trip down Grandma Road… I'm never coming back!

Father, thank you for your faithfulness, your unfailing love, and for keeping your promises forever. Thank you for your tender mercies and the precious gift of new life. Amen.

51

REAL LOVE

God showed how much he loved us by sending his only Son into the world so that we might have eternal life through him. This is real love. It is not that we loved God, but that he loved us and sent his Son as a sacrifice to take away our sins. — 1 John 4:9-10

"God loves you." These three words are among the first words I usually speak to people who come to me for ministry after a cancer diagnosis. I can always see the doubt in their eyes. "God loves me? How could that be?" A diagnosis of cancer can make even the most devout person begin to doubt the nature of God. It can be tempting to wonder if He's given up on us, He's punishing us, or He simply doesn't care. It's important to know that the cancer you battled did not come from God. Jesus did not come to condemn steal, kill, or destroy. He came to give full and abundant life (John 10:10). Satan was the culprit behind the cancer that tried to destroy you. He makes it his business to prowl around like a roaring lion looking for some unsuspecting victim to devour (1 Peter 5:8).

In contrast, God's nature is to love. God *is* love (1 John 4:8). He created you out of love and you are perfectly and wonderfully made, a precious masterpiece in His eyes (Psalm 139:14; Ephesians 2:10). His love for you knows no boundaries (Hosea 14:4). To help you grasp the concept of infinite love, just imagine standing on a beach with the sandy shoreline extending for miles and miles on each side. You reach down and scoop up a handful of sand. As the grains of sand slowly run through your fingers, think about this: His thoughts about you far outnumber the grains of sand on the entire beach (Psalm 139:17-18). Now gaze at the vast ocean in front of you, and imagine His love stretching out as far as the eye can see. It's wide enough to cover the sorrows of today and long enough to cover your uncertain tomorrows. His love reaches up as high as the heavens are above the water and as deep as the ocean floor. It touches the heights of your good times and the depths of your despair (Ephesians 3:17-19). There is nothing — not death or life, not angels or demons, not our fears for today or our worries about tomorrow, not the powers of hell, not cancer — that can ever keep His love away from you (Romans 8:38).

From the depths of His love, God cares for you. He delights in your company (Psalm 18:19). He takes great joy in every minute you can find to spend with Him. He has compassion for the sick and the hurting (Matthew 14:14). He is a merciful God who comforts you with His strength, encouragement, and hope (2 Corinthians 1:3). He wept along with you when the bad news came (John 11:34-36). There is no condemnation in Him when you fall short (Romans 8:1). He understands how weak you are (Psalm 103:14).

In the aftermath of cancer, we can be tempted to allow disappointment and weariness cause us to doubt God's love. We might even let our past experiences with an earthly father or authority figure cloud our view of the nature of God. If you are a parent and you are struggling to accept God's love for you, let me ask you a question: Would you strike your own children with a devastating disease and then abandon them in the middle of nowhere as a punishment for their misbehavior? If your children asked you for a loaf of bread, would you give them a stone? If they asked you for a fish, would you give them a snake? Jesus said if we sinful and fallible people know how to give good gifts to our children, then how much more will our heavenly Father give to us (Matthew 7:9-11)?

God is not cruel, vindictive, or indifferent. He is a loving Father who understands and cares for you, infinitely more so than the best earthly parent. His proved His love by sacrificing His own Son for the sins of the world. Jesus chose you first (John 15:16). He suffered and died, rose again, and extended the invitation for you to join Him forever in eternity. He allows you to make the next choice; to except or reject His divine love offering. Don't let anything stand in the way of your decision. His love is unconditional, unfailing, infinite, and real.

Father, thank you for your Son and the gift of eternal life. Forgive me for doubting your love. Help me to understand your nature and truly grasp the width, length, height, and depth of your love for me. Amen.

52

True Humility

True humility and fear of the LORD lead to riches, honor, and long life. — Proverbs 22:4

I spend a lot of time on a motorcycle, but my husband does all the driving. This summer I learned it should probably stay that way. At our annual Hosanna! Biker ministry retreat, one of the guys brought a Yamaha 50 mini-bike to ride around the camp. Everyone was taking turns and they finally convinced me to give it a try. I had never driven a motorcycle before, but how hard could it be? It was a kid bike! I got on and with everyone gathered around watching, I circled around the camp. I was quite proud of myself and all the cheering and shouts of "Do it again!" easily swayed me. My second run didn't work out so well. This time, instead of making the corner, I crashed head on into a building — a church no less. It was scene readymade for America's Funniest Videos. Unfortunately, it was caught on video and played repeatedly for the rest of the weekend. I was a perfect advertisement for the well known Proverb, "pride goes before a fall."

Pride is at the root of every sin. It came into humankind in the Garden when Satan convinced Adam and Eve if they ate from the Tree of Knowledge they could be like God. Pride manifests through a variety of ungodly mindsets. I can believe I'm right and everyone else is wrong, when the truth is that everyone is created in God's image and has a unique set of life experiences and beliefs. I can isolate myself and believe that depending on people leads to weakness when the truth is that God created me to live in community as part of the Body of Christ. I can believe that I don't need God when the truth is I am completely dependent on Him for my every breath. I can believe my appearance and performance will earn love, respect, and status, when the truth is my true identity is in Christ. Sometimes pride drives the most devout of church-goers. There are people who habitually manipulate conversations with "God told me…," making it very difficult to disagree with a direct word from the Lord. Some have an elevated view their denomination, some go to church to make an appearance, while others boast about their church's superior worship style, music, or preaching.

The exact opposite of pride is humility. In our attempts to be humble, we can have false humility. When I compliment someone on a job well done and they say, "Oh, it wasn't me, it was God," I want to say, "Well, if God did it, it would have been much better!" Sometimes people give the appearance of humility by putting their own needs aside simply to manipulate others. There is nothing humble about putting yourself down to others, especially when the underlying motive is to gain their disagreement with your criticism and elicit compliments.

Jesus taught about true humility when He noticed all who were coming for dinner were vying for a seat at head of the table. Instead, He advises them to sit at the foot of the table and allow the host to honor them in front of all the guests by inviting them to a better seat, "for the proud will be humbled, but the humble will be honored" (Luke 14:7-11). Jesus also said anyone who becomes as humble as a little child is the greatest in the Kingdom of Heaven (Matthew 18:4). The disciples had become so pre-occupied with organizing around the ministry of Jesus and jockeying for status and position that they lost sight of their divine purpose. True humility comes from knowing that greatness comes from serving, not focusing on self. True humility is comparing ourselves with Christ and recognizing our sinfulness and limitations and our need for Him. It is recognizing our gifts and strengths and serving according to His will.

Jesus is the perfect example of humility. He humbled Himself in Heaven by giving up His rights as God and coming to earth in human form. He humbled Himself on earth by going willingly to the cross to die a criminal's death. Because of this, God lifted Him up to the highest place of honor (Philippians 2:7-9). He will do the same for you, and you don't have to crash into any buildings in the process. Humble yourself under His mighty power and He will lift you up (1 Peter 5:6). With long life, He will honor you.

Father, thank you for your Son Jesus, the perfect example of true humility. Help me to see where I have let pride enter my life. Help me to become as humble as a little child by recognizing my total dependence on you alone. Amen.

53

THE PATH OF BLESSING

You know these things — now do them! That is the path of blessing.
— John 13:17

A few years ago, our church sent a mission team to India to share the hope of the Gospel. Even though I had been to Sri Lanka and several other under-developed countries, nothing prepared me for the sights, sounds, and smells of India. From the moment the doors of the plane opened, my heart broke for the people and the seemingly infinite chasm between their need and the world's resources. But we had come with an answer — we brought Jesus, the hope of all the world. The local pastors and church leaders had made painstaking plans for our visit and honored us as we taught, worshipped, and prayed for them in preparation for the four-day evangelistic campaign we would co-lead for the public.

I will never forget the day when the leaders of our group washed the feet of the leaders of theirs. Our desire was to build unity and to show the full extent of our love. Tears streamed down my cheeks, mingling with the water I was pouring over the feet of a woman wearing a beautiful red sari. When I finished, I dried her feet, set the basin aside and embraced her. As I buried my head in her shoulders, her tears spilled out onto my hair. She was overwhelmed with the love of Jesus, and I was overwhelmed with love and the privilege of serving Him.

On the night before His death, Jesus laid out the path of blessing. He got up from the table, took off His robe, and wrapped it around His waist. He then proceeded to wash the disciples' feet and dry them with a towel (John 13:1-5). In this culture, washing the feet of a house guest was the task of a lowly servant. But Jesus had no problem humbling Himself in this role. He knew His identity and that He had authority over all things. He knew He came from the Father and would return to the Father. Peter didn't understand (John 13:6). In his world view, leaders were supposed to lead, and servants were supposed to serve. Jesus explained His actions this way: "Since I, the Lord and Teacher, have washed your feet, you ought to wash other's feet. I have given an example to follow. Do as I have done to you" (John 13:14-15). Jesus was giving instructions to extend His mission to earth after He was gone. These men were to go into the world to serve God, each other, and all those people who needed to hear the Good News.

This same message extends to us. If God in the flesh is willing to serve, His followers must also be willing to serve in any way that glorifies God, because "a servant is not greater than the master" (John 13:16). It is one thing to know and believe that humble service is the way of Jesus, but quite another to actually serve Him. I have to admit, washing the feet of this Indian woman stretched me way out of my comfort zone. But the blessing that came from this humble act of service was beyond anything I could imagine. My discomfort was soon forgotten as I experienced the overwhelming presence of Jesus. We were in God's perfect will and acted out of pure obedience. We followed His example. As a result, the entire team of Indian pastors was anointed and empowered to step into their leadership role as servants of Jesus in this part of India. Thousands of people have come to the Lord because of their ministry.

In the same way, God will stretch you. He will ask you to follow His example. You may have to go against the world's perspective and take the position of a humble servant. When you know what He wants you to do, take the next step. Do it. That is the path of blessing.

Father, thank you for the example of your servant Jesus. Please stretch me so that I may act in obedience and live a life of humble service that brings you glory. Amen.

54

CITIZENS OF HEAVEN

But we are citizens of heaven, where the Lord Jesus Christ lives.
And we are eagerly waiting for him to return as our Savior.
— Philippians 3:20

Jan is a poster child for the fruit of the spirit. Love, joy, peace, patience, kindness, goodness, faithfulness, gentleness and self-control flow out of her like a river (Galatians 5:22-23). When Jan was diagnosed with Stage 3 colon cancer, her doctors gave her a 20 percent chance to survive. That was over 14 years ago. She's still surviving and thriving and the fruit is still flowing. Jan loves life and lives it to its fullest. Her joy and passion are infectious. Everyone she encounters walks away with an extra spring in their step. They're not sure what she has or what she's on, but they want a dose of it.

What's her secret? Many would say there is no logical earthly reason why someone like Jan should be so downright cheerful. But Jan is not of this world. She is a foreigner just passing through a world that would prefer to keep God at a distance (1 Peter 2:11). She is a citizen of Heaven where the Lord Jesus Christ lives. She knows that Heaven is not some pink cloud-in-the-sky existence she hopes to enjoy someday in the future. The Kingdom of Heaven is already here! It arrived on earth in the person of Jesus Christ. It spread throughout the entire world when the Holy Spirit came to live and rule in the hearts of every believer. And someday when Jesus comes back and God judges and destroys all sin, the Kingdom of Heaven will rule every corner of the earth (Revelation 21:3).

Just like you and me, Jan is a weak and fallible human being, struggling to travel through a life filled with unexpected twists and turns. But her decision to make the Kingdom of Heaven her home on earth has made all the difference. Nothing in her outward behavior comes from her own strength and abilities. The character traits in her that people admire and covet come from more than a positive attitude or a sunny disposition. They are character traits found in the very nature of Christ. They are produced by the power of the Holy Spirit as a result of letting Christ control her life.

When God has His rightful place in the center of your life, the light and power of the Holy Spirit can't help but shine within and through you, regardless of the trials you are experiencing (2 Corinthians 4:7). A transformed life and an attitude that defies all the world's expectations are effective testimony to the power of God (Philippians 2:14-15). People will see all that love, joy, and peace flowing out of you and know immediately something is different about you. They'll be curious and want what you have. And you can tell them. "This world is not my home. I'm a citizen of Heaven where the Lord Jesus Christ lives."

Father, thank you that by the death and resurrection of your Son, I am a citizen of Heaven. Help me to make your Kingdom my home on earth. Let your light shine through me! Amen.

55

BUCKTHORN ATTACK

"Your eye is a lamp that provides light for your body.
When your eye is good, your whole body is filled with light.
But when your eye is bad, your whole body is filled with darkness.
And if the light you think you have is actually darkness,
how deep that darkness is!" — Matthew 6:22-23

It was Thanksgiving weekend. The weather was unseasonably warm and the Christmas lights were successfully hung on the house when my husband got motivated to remove the buckthorns in our densely wooded backyard. Buckthorns are invasive shrubs or small trees that have become a serious problem in Minnesota's woodlands because they crowd out native plants. His timing was perfect. Fall is the easiest time to identify buckthorns because their leaves don't change color until most of the other trees have already dropped their leaves. Buckthorns have low branches with nasty thorns, making removal difficult and even a walk through the woods unpleasant. He learned the hard way just how unpleasant they can be. With his chainsaw roaring, he attacked his prey with a vengeance as the buckthorns fell in droves. He was tugging at one particularly stubborn plant, when the plant struck back. One of its thorny branches snapped back and whipped him in the face, sending his eye glasses sailing through the woods. I wasn't home at the time, so he had no choice but to grope blindly for his glasses on his own. He searched the woods for an hour without success.

Sometimes life is a lot like my like my husband's encounter with buckthorn. It can snap back, whip you in the face, and plunge you into darkness! Darkness creeps into our soul when we take our eyes off Jesus, the source of all light. Sometimes our circumstances distract us. Peter had great faith when he jumped out of the boat and walked on water until he took his eyes off Jesus and focused on the high waves around him (Matthew 14:28-29). If we focus on our problems and circumstances instead looking to Jesus in faith, we can easily despair and sink into darkness.

Unrepented sin can also pull our focus off Jesus, plunge us into moral darkness, and cut us off from God. We can become so focused on our own self-interests, desires, and goals that we lose our sense of values. Obsessing over money, possessions, hobbies, and temporal things makes us blind to eternal things. We can be lost without any concept of where we're going. The prophet Isaiah vividly describes the consequences of a lifestyle of unrepented sin: "So there is no justice among us, and we know nothing about right living. We look for light but find only darkness. We look for bright skies but walk in gloom. We grope like the blind along a wall, feeling our way like people without eyes. Even at brightest noontime, we stumble as though it were dark" (Isaiah 59: 9-10).

My husband never found his glasses. Fortunately, he found an old pair to wear until he could order a new pair. He experienced a practical reminder of the importance of clear vision to help us see what we're doing and where we're going. In the same way, clear spiritual vision gives heavenly purposes and desires to our earthly life. What is pulling you away from God today? What is tempting to plunge you into darkness? Whatever it might be, Jesus came to rescue you! He called you out of the darkness into His wonderful light (1 Peter 2:9). When you fix your eyes on Him, He floods your whole body with light so you can understand the wonderful future He has promised to those He called (Ephesians 1:18). His truth, penetrating into your heart, brings life and radiant health to your body (Proverbs 4:21-22). Stay in His glorious light. No mistake is too great for Him to forgive and no problem too big for Him to handle. The next time the buckthorn attacks, you'll be ready.

Father, thank you for sending your Son to rescue me from the darkness. Help me to keep my eyes focused on you, Jesus. I want to live in your light! Amen.

56

Broken Bones

Give all your worries and cares to God, for he cares about you.
— 1 Peter 5:7

Last night, my two-year old grandson broke his leg. He took a nasty fall on the living room floor and fractured his tibia. Imagine an active toddler immobilized for at least six weeks in a cast with a brand new baby sister. My heart aches for him and his parents. I'm always amazed by my reaction when my children or grandchildren are suffering. My "mother bear" instinct takes over and I want to fix it. I want to step in and take over. I want to protect them from this evil world and everything that could possibly hurt them. Essentially, I want to play God. All of these things are His job, not mine. My job is to pray. And to give him lots of Grandma hugs.

Whenever we worry about our problems and carry the responsibility for fixing them on our own shoulders, we are not trusting God with the details of our lives. The Apostle Paul offers an alternative. He instructs us to turn our worries into prayers. If we pray about everything and thank God for all He has done, He promises to give us a peace that surpasses all human understanding (Philippians 4:6-7). This peace does not depend on circumstances, the absence of problems, or good feelings. It comes from knowing

God is still on the throne and has won the victory over sin and death and every problem we will ever face, including a little boy with a broken leg.

We are especially tempted to carry burdens on our own shoulders if we blame ourselves and believe our problems have originated from our own mistakes. We hesitate to turn to God in prayer because we think He won't have compassion on us to help. But His love is unfailing and His tender mercies start fresh every day. If we turn to Him in repentance, He bears the weight of any struggle we will ever encounter. Instead of submitting to our circumstances, we can submit to the Lord who is sovereign over all our circumstances, regardless of the cause.

When I think of my grandson, I'm reminded of a verse in the Psalms: "For the Lord protects the bones of the righteous; not one of them is broken" (Psalm 34:20)! The meaning of this verse is twofold; first, it is a prophesy about Jesus. Not one of His bones was broken to speed his sacrificial death on the cross, even though it was Roman custom at the time. But it is also a verse proclaiming that we can trust God for protection in times of trouble. Sometimes He rescues us from imminent danger, and other times He carries us safely through it. Our little guy may have a broken leg, but we can trust God, not Grandma or even his parents, to be his true source of power and strength. We can trust God to heal his leg and comfort his spirit. And we can trust Him to redeem every minute of his pain and suffering.

No matter how broken you may be today, He will do the same for you. Perhaps you carry the burden of worry for a loved one on your shoulders, or maybe some problems in your own life feel insurmountable. Maybe you are simply weary of the physical or emotional effects that remain, even after cancer has left your body. Whatever your circumstances might be, turn your worries into prayers, and receive His perfect peace. Trust in God alone to fix your problems. Give all your worries and cares to Him. He really does care about you.

Father, thank you for doing the heavy lifting and carrying all the weight of my problems on your shoulders. Help me to turn my worries into prayers and trust you with the details of my life. Amen.

57

Seek First His Kingdom

Seek the Kingdom of God above all else, and live righteously, and he will give you everything you need. — Matthew 6:33

Margie had just finished treatment for stage 3 uterine cancer. She had barely regained her strength and was recovering from the emotional and physical trauma when her husband suffered a serious injury at work that required multiple surgeries. Margie had missed so much work from her own treatment that they were already struggling to make ends meet. Now, they had to wait until his worker's compensation benefits became effective. In the meantime, their bills wouldn't wait. When they came to the church for help, they were blessed to receive some financial assistance to tide them over.

I have a similar story. Eight months after I had finished treatment for breast cancer and I was just getting re-established in my consulting practice, my husband lost his job. He was the primary income source for our family and carried the health insurance through his company. We had just finished educating our son, our daughter was a freshman in college, and my cancer history made buying private health insurance impossible. My husband was unemployed for 14 months. I'm always amazed at

God's faithfulness during this time. It cost over $1000 a month to extend his work sponsored healthcare plan through COBRA in addition to all our other living expenses. Somehow, between the unemployment benefits and my consulting income, we managed to make ends meet.

In these tough economic times, many people are struggling, even without the challenges of cancer. You may find yourself in a similar position. You may be celebrating the healing God gave you, while at the same time, wondering how you will pay the mortgage, your healthcare bills, or meet the basic needs of your family. The good news is that God cares about those who depend on Him. Jesus made it very clear that we don't have to worry about the needs of everyday life. The same God who created you can be trusted with the details of sustaining you. He feeds the birds that don't plant, harvest, or store up food, and you are far more valuable to Him than birds. If He clothes beautiful flowers that are here today and gone tomorrow, He will certainly care for you. It may come as a surprise to you, but God already knows all of your needs (Matthew 25:32)!

There is nothing fruitful or positive about worry, especially during times of waiting when the answers are unclear. Nothing good will come from it. It can damage your health, distract you from your work and leisure for today, and keep you from trusting God to meet your needs. Jesus gives us the perfect antidote for worry. Seek first His Kingdom. Put Him first in your life. Fill your thoughts with His desires, not yours. Make Him first on your priority list before people, money, possessions, and personal goals. Seek Him first, before mortgage payments, healthcare bills, food, clothing, or any other basic needs. When the stresses and strains of everyday living creep in and try to bump Him out, choose God, not worry. Worry immobilizes, but seeking God through prayer and His Word gives wisdom, direction, purpose, and clarity.

There is a wonderful promise attached to this Scripture; if you do these things and live righteously, He will give you everything you need. He did it for Margie, He did it for me, and He will do it for you. Seek first His Kingdom.

Father, thank you for the promise to provide for all of my needs. Help me not to worry. Help me to seek you first. Amen.

58

LOVE CAME DOWN

The Word became human and lived among us. — John 1:14

I've been blessed to have celebrated many Christmases in my life. I won't tell you exactly how many, but lots! The older I get, the faster time passes. It feels like I just take the Christmas tree down, and it's time to put it back up again. As I reflect on the years gone by, I have to admit I experienced my first real Christmas in 1999. This was the Christmas I finally "got it." I was at the Christmas Eve worship service halfway through my chemo treatments and wearing a wig to cover my bald head when our worship leader sang, "Emmanuel, God is With Us." The words pierced my heart. *God is with us.* The same God who created the heavens and earth, set the stars in place and called them by name, came to earth as a humble baby. Love came down. I couldn't wrap my mind around a God who would give up His rights as God and make Himself nothing; a God who would take the humble position of a slave and appear on earth in human form (Philippians 2:6-7).

Why would He do such a thing? God sent His Son to earth to restore what Satan stole in the Garden of Eden. It was always His intention to live in intimate relationship with us, but after the "fall," mankind was banished from His presence. From that point on, generation after generation of people repeatedly turned their hearts away from God to follow their sinful nature, even though He extended His mercy countless times. By the time Jesus came, the Jews were hopelessly oppressed by the Roman Empire, desperately waiting for their long awaited Messiah to come to establish a new kingdom and rule the world with justice.

They had good reason for hope. Over 300 prophesies said He would come to save them. Micah foretold of a Ruler who will "stand and lead His flock with the Lord's strength, in the majesty of the name of the Lord his God," and He will be the source of our peace" (Micah 5:4,5). The prophet Isaiah said the people who walk in darkness will see a great light — a light that will shine on all who live in the land where death casts its shadow (Isaiah 9:2). He prophesied the mission of Jesus when He said: "The Spirit of the Sovereign Lord is upon me, for the Lord has anointed me to bring good news to the poor. He has sent me to comfort the brokenhearted and to proclaim that captives will be released and prisoners will be freed" (Isaiah 61:1).

The ministry of Jesus officially began when he visited the synagogue in His boyhood home of Nazareth and read the prophetic words of Isaiah that He had come to heal the brokenhearted, release the captives, restore sight to the blind, and free the downtrodden from their oppressors (Luke 4:18). Then He added: "The Scripture you've just heard has been fulfilled this very day" (Luke 4:21)! But this was not His only purpose for coming. After He destroyed sin's control over us by sacrificing His life on the cross, He sent the Holy Spirit to restore the relationship we had with Him in the Garden by dwelling in each believer.

This year, like every year, I'll enjoy choosing special gifts for my loved ones and carefully wrapping them in beautiful paper and ribbons to put under the tree. With each package I wrap, I never forget that the first gift wrap was swaddling clothes. There are many things you might want for Christmas this year, but there is only one thing you truly need. Jesus satisfies every want and need you will ever have. The best Christmas present you will ever receive is the privilege of living in His "presence." Love came down. Receive the gift!

Father, thank you for a love so great I will never fully understand it. You gave up your rights as God to save me! Help me to receive the precious gift of your presence. Amen.

59

SECOND OPINION

*Trust in the LORD with all your heart; do not depend on
your own understanding. Seek his will in all you do, and he will
direct your paths.* — Proverbs 3:5-6

It was John's first time at Pray for the Cure, the healing ministry
I lead at our church. He made his way through a group of people
mingling near the entrance of the prayer chapel and found a
seat among the circle of chairs. While others carried on friendly
conversation as they waited for the prayer meeting to begin, John
was silent. He was well-dressed and distinguished looking; clearly
a man of significance who has known success. Yet, there was an air
of humility about him.

After I prayed, John listened attentively to those gathered around
the circle to receive prayers of healing for themselves or their loved
ones. Four young women undergoing breast cancer treatment each
shared their story. One had just finished radiation, another was
beginning chemo, and the rest were in the midst of it. They laughed
and compared side effects as they candidly shared their fears and
concerns with the group. An older gentleman accompanied by his
wife and daughter struggled to tell his recent diagnosis of advanced
pancreatic cancer. He was apprehensive about starting chemo the next

day. A 10-year survivor of lymphoma shared his journey of faith. A man in a wheelchair explained the events leading up to his diagnosis and his first chemo treatment for abdominal carcinosarcoma. His wife held his hand while fighting back tears.

It was John's turn to share. A five-year survivor of prostate cancer, John had received a full course of treatment and an optimistic prognosis. At his annual checkup last week, he learned that his PSA score had suddenly risen. His doctor wanted to start treatment immediately. John wasn't sure. Something deep in his spirit told him to wait. He needed time to think and pray. In church that Sunday, he saw a bulletin announcement for Pray for the Cure and felt a tugging in his heart to attend the next evening. In obedience, John had come to seek God's direction. He had come for prayer.

When we gathered around John for prayer that evening, we thanked God for the gift of John's healing. We prayed for wisdom and clarity, for both John and his doctor. John gave the test results to God and trusted He would provide discernment. We asked God to direct John's path of decision-making. We prayed for the peace that surpasses all human understanding. We asked God to guard his heart against doubt and anxiety.

John left that night without a clear course of action, but completely confident that God would show his faithfulness. The next month, he came back to the prayer meeting to share his wonderful news. When he had returned to the doctor for retesting, the PSA was back to normal. Subsequent tests showed the same amazing result. His doctor would continue monitoring, but John's PSA is normal — no need for treatment. We prayed again, but this time, we joined John in a prayer of praise and gratitude and asked for the Lord's continued protection.

John knew God healed him and made it perfectly clear through the PSA score that no treatment was necessary. He had sought the Lord with all His heart. He didn't depend solely on his own understanding or the counsel of his doctor. He invited God into the entire situation and surrendered leadership to Him. And God was faithful.

It may not come naturally to seek a second opinion when such urgent counsel comes from a trusted doctor, especially one who has cared for us through the trauma of a cancer diagnosis. But God knows our needs better than anyone. He will provide for us from day to day if we choose to give him first place in every area of our lives (Matthew 6:33). Trusting Him doesn't mean we should ignore God-given human wisdom. It simply means we shouldn't trust our own understanding or the counsel of wise doctors at the exclusion of God. Seek his opinion in all your medical decisions. Let His Word guide you and follow His leading. If you do, He promises to protect you and direct your paths.

Father, thank you for your faithfulness and your continued protection over my health. Help me to not lean on my human understanding, but to trust you with all my heart. Amen.

60

No Plan B

And Jesus said to him, "Go your way. Your faith has healed you." And instantly the blind man could see! — Mark 10:52

A few years ago, I was privileged to be part of an evangelism campaign in the city of Amednagar, India. Most of the crowd that gathered under the stadium lights had heard about Jesus, a Healer, who lived long ago and was raised from the dead. In the weeks before, billboards throughout the town encouraged them to come and learn more about Him. They came because He was their only hope. There were few doctors and no money to pay them. Most were "untouchables," born into the lowest class of a caste system that banned them from full participation in Hindu social life. They were held captive to a life of discrimination, poverty, and unrestrained violence with no hope of escape. At the campaign, they learned that Jesus loved them. In His Kingdom, everyone was equal. Rich or poor, untouchable or not, His followers all shared the same eternal future. They learned Jesus could meet their every need. Over the course of four days, people streamed into the stadium and waited for their turn on the prayer line. We prayed and God healed. The mutes could speak, the blind could see, the deaf could hear, and the lame could walk, just as in the early church.

As I wonder why there were so many miraculous healings in India and not back home, I'm convinced of one thing: in India, there is no Plan B. In our culture, we can pray for a headache at church on Sunday and go to the doctor on Monday. For many people in countries like India, there are no doctors accessible to them if the prayers "don't work."

Bartemaeus, the blind beggar, had no Plan B. His blindness forced him to beg along with others like him who had disabilities that made it impossible for them to make an honest living. The people had long ago forgotten God's law that they should care for them. Instead, blindness was considered a curse from God for sin. One day, as Bartemaeus sat along the road on the way to Jericho, he heard that Jesus of Nazareth was passing by. He instantly began shouting, "Jesus, Son of David, have mercy on me!" The crowd ahead of Jesus tried to hush him but he only shouted louder. He persisted until Jesus stopped and ordered that he be brought to Him. Recklessly throwing down his coat, he jumped up and rushed over to Jesus. "What do you want me to do for you?" asked Jesus. Bartemaeus shouted in reply, "Lord, I want to see!" Jesus said, "Go your way, your faith has healed you." Instantly he could see (Mark 10:46-52).

Just as the people we ministered to in India, Bartemaeus had little hope of escaping his situation, but he had hope in Jesus. By calling Him "Son of David," Bartemaeus acknowledged Him as the long awaited Messiah the Scriptures foretold would be a descendent of King David (Isaiah 9:7). He shamelessly called out for Jesus' attention in spite of the crowd's rebuke. Without thinking, he threw down his coat — most likely his only possession — to come to Jesus and tell Him what he wanted. He was determined not to let Jesus pass him by without receiving his healing. His reckless faith allowed him to see.

Bartamaeus, a blind man, recognized Jesus as the long awaited Messiah, while the religious leaders of his day watched Him perform countless miracles and were blind to his identity. The people in India had only heard that Jesus heals. They had no reason to doubt what they had heard. They weren't hindered by religious traditions and didn't need to solve all the mysteries of God's ways in order to believe. Don't let Him pass by without opening your eyes. He is the Son of David, your Savior and King! Pursue Him with a reckless hope. Pursue Him like there's no Plan B.

Father, thank you for sending Jesus, the Healer of all my diseases. Don't let Him pass me by. Give me a reckless faith. I want to see! Amen.

61

STAY GREEN

"Yes, I am the vine; you are the branches. Those who remain in me, and I in them, will produce much fruit. For apart from me you can do nothing. — John 15:5

I love spending the weekend after Thanksgiving decorating for Christmas. It beats fighting the crowds on Black Friday. This year, I wanted to do something different on my kitchen table, so I went to the local nursery and bought a fresh silver fir wreath. It was healthy, green and, better yet, on sale! The guy at the nursery warned me it might not last long inside. He suggested I keep it outside and bring it in closer to Christmas. But I had a table to decorate. I ignored his advice, set the wreath on a beautiful red tapestry runner, and placed a hurricane lamp in the middle with a red candle inside. Then, I proceeded to decorate the wreath with pinecones and holly berries. The entire centerpiece was beautiful. I thought for sure if I sprayed the wreath with water a couple times a day, it would surely stay green until Christmas. Not so. Five days later, my masterpiece was turning brown. Ten days later, it was as good as dead.

My wreath turned brown and died because it was made from branches that had been cut from the silver fir tree, it's only source of water and sustenance. It reminds me that Christ is the vine and we, as followers, are the branches. Father God is the Gardener who takes care of us and makes us fruitful. If we stay connected to Jesus, the vine, we'll stay green and bear much fruit. But if we are separated, we turn brown and fruitless like the wreath on my table. We can try to feel alive by pursuing possessions, busyness, adventure, and the values of the world. We can even be convinced that staying emotionally and physically well is completely dependent on our doctors, our knowledge, our habits, and our own strengths. But we are really doing nothing more than spraying water on the wreath in hopes of keeping it green. There is no sustainable life giving power without Jesus. We can do nothing without Him. We can't bear fruit that lasts. If we're not careful about remaining in Jesus, sooner or later, we can find ourselves spiritually as good as dead.

Remaining in Jesus is more than believing He is who He says He is and receiving Him as Lord and Savior. All of this is important, but remaining in Him is a two way street; the Scripture says, "those who remain in me, and I in them…" When we become believers, He comes to dwell in us through the powerful presence of the Holy Spirit. We remain in Him through obedience to His Word (1 John 3:24), by continuing to be faithful to what we have been taught (1 John 2:24), and by loving others as Christ loves us (John 15:12). He is always present and waiting to fellowship with us. When we yield to His Spirit within us, we are compelled to stay in fellowship with Him through reading His Word, prayer, or simply resting in His presence. We can't go weeks, months, or even days without connecting with Jesus, anymore than my wreath can stay green without being connected to its life source.

Intimacy with Jesus produces fruit that lasts — spiritual blessings for yourself as well as for those around you. Jesus said if you will stay joined to Him and His words remain in you, you will receive the blessing of answered prayer (John 15:7). You will experience overflowing joy regardless of your circumstances (John 15:11). Your interactions with others and the world around you will be marked by your love, joy, peace, patience, kindness, goodness, faithfulness, gentleness, and self-control (Galatians 5:22-23). All of this is yours because you stay connected to the One true vine. Apart from Him, you can do nothing that really lasts. There is no life-giving power without Him. There is no other way to truly stay green.

Father, thank you for taking care of me and making me fruitful. Help me to stay connected to Jesus and so I can bear lasting fruit for your Kingdom. Amen.

62

The Secret Place

Those who live in the shelter of the Most High will find rest in the shadow of the Almighty. This I declare of the LORD: He alone is my refuge, my place of safety; he is my God, and I am trusting him. If you make the LORD your refuge, if you make the Most High your shelter, no evil will conquer you; no plague will come near your dwelling. — Psalm 91:1-2, 9-10

Before I entered the ministry and even before I started my consulting practice, I held a high level management position in a major corporation. The job was incredibly stressful, so much so that I would occasionally suffer panic attacks. I learned later that people having panic attacks experience a type of "fight or flight" response, the same physical symptoms as someone in immediate physical danger. Once this response kicks in, we tend to perceive everything around us as a potential safety threat. When this happened, I would always retreat to my office and read Psalm 91. I was not very Bible literate at the time, but reading this Psalm always took me to a secret place with God when I found myself paralyzed with fear. I learned I could go to Him for protection and trade my fear for peace. Regardless of how crazy things got, I could rest in Him and trust Him to keep me safe. As a reminder of God's protection for me and all who enter my home, these verses are beautifully framed on the wall in my entry way.

The author of Psalm 91 refers my secret place as "the shadow," "my refuge," "my place of safety," "shelter" and "dwelling." Other Psalmists like those below describe my secret place as "my hiding place," "shadow of your wings," "shelter of your wings," a "fortress," and "sanctuary:"

• For you are my hiding place; you protect me from trouble. You surround me with songs of victory (Psalm 32:7).

• How precious is your unfailing love, O God! All humanity finds shelter in the shadow of your wings (Psalm 36:7).

• The LORD saves the godly; he is their fortress in times of trouble. The LORD helps them, rescuing them from the wicked. He saves them, and they find shelter in him (Psalm 37:39-40).

• Have mercy on me, O God, have mercy! I look to you for protection. I will hide beneath the shadow of your wings until this violent storm is past (Psalm 57:1).

• Lead me to the towering rock of safety, for you are my safe refuge, a fortress where my enemies cannot reach me. Let me live forever in your sanctuary, safe beneath the shelter of your wings (Psalm 61:2-4)!

David directly refers to being hidden "in the secret place of your presence" and being kept "secretly in a pavilion" (Psalm 31:20,

NKJV). Jesus came to make the secret place of God's presence accessible to everyone who believes. He made it clear when he announced that "the Kingdom of God is near" (Mark 1:15)! The long awaited Messiah had come to break the power of sin and begin God's reign on earth. He came to bring the Good News of the Kingdom by teaching, preaching, and healing people of every kind of disease and sickness (Mark 4:23). The Kingdom is not just a future place, but a realm of power today. In this secret place, under God's divine rule and reign, and by the power of the Holy Spirit, there is freedom, hope, peaceful living, abundant life, and eternal joy.

Yes, there is still evil in the world. Jesus said we will have many trials and sorrows on earth, but to take heart, because He has overcome the world. We can have peace in Him (John 16:33). Until He returns, He gave us the Holy Spirit as foretaste future glory — a time when God will completely free the world of all sin, sickness, and evil (Romans 8:19-23). In the meantime, God is with us. We can hide in His presence until the violent storms pass. He promises shelter for the oppressed and refuge in times of trouble (Psalm 9:9).

In Scripture often read at funerals, Jesus tells His disciples not to let their hearts be troubled because He is going to prepare a place for them (John 14:1-2). Just as He has prepared an eternal place for you in Heaven, He has prepared a special place for you right here on earth. In His presence, you will find protection from harm, rest for your soul, and the courage to face your fears. The next time trouble sends you into a panic, trade all your fears for a supernatural peace that surpasses human understanding. Make the Most High your shelter, and no evil will conquer you. Meet Him in the secret place.

Father, thank you for the promise of your presence. Please protect me in your secret place when trouble threatens to come. Keep me safe beneath the shadow of your wings. Amen.

63

SALTY FLATS

*They are like stunted shrubs in the desert, with no hope
for the future. They will live in the barren wilderness, on the salty
flats where no one lives.* — Jeremiah 17:6

We have logged over 75,000 miles on our Gold Wing motorcycle, and most of these miles have been cross country. My favorite trip was our very first on the bike. We road across the plains of North Dakota, through the Big Horn Mountains of Wyoming, up north through Montana to Glacier National Park, and across Washington state. We ferried our bikes up to Vancouver BC, took the coast highway down to San Francisco, and then circled back home on a northeasterly route to Minnesota. It was 16 days and 5316 miles of shear breathtaking beauty, with a few of noteworthy exceptions. With all due respect to the people of Utah, I could have lived without going through the Bonneville Salt Flats. There was nothing there but flat desert ground covered with densely packed salt as far as the eye could see. It was over a hundred degrees, and we drove for about 40 miles without so much as a gas station. At the one rest stop, we gratefully pumped undrinkable water from a well to soak our clothing and cool off. And the "facilities?" Let's just say it was preferable to wait.

I can see why people go there to race their cars and motorcycles. I can also see why few people live in this hopeless, barren, salty land. It reminded me of the empty spiritual existence experienced by those who put their trust in mere humans instead of God, and turn their hearts away from Him (Jeremiah 17:5).

On the same trip, we drove through the Colorado River valley where there were lush green trees lining the riverbank through miles and miles of canyon. What a contrast to the salt flats! The prophet Jeremiah used the analogy of trees planted along a riverbank with roots that reach deep into the water to describe those who trust in the Lord and have made the Him their hope and confidence. The leaves of these trees stay green, and they go right on producing delicious fruit even during long stretches of heat or draught (Jeremiah 17:7-8).

When you turned to the Lord in your cancer crisis, your roots of faith grew deeper. As He guided you safely through the desert to the other side, your roots continued to press downward into the soil of His love. Now, as you continue to make the Lord your hope and confidence, He will become more and more at home in your heart, and your roots will penetrate even deeper (Ephesians 3:17). With a deeply rooted faith, you will no longer be moved by your circumstances. The doctor visits and checkups that follow cancer treatment can be stressful, but you won't have to wilt with worry. You won't have to panic if they have to repeat a mammogram to get a better shot or leave you waiting for the phone to ring. Regardless of the next crisis you face, regardless of the season of life you find yourself in, your leaves will stay green.

A deeply rooted faith comes from building your life on Jesus and His Word and relying on Him to carry you through, from one trial to the next. As He shows His faithfulness and your faith grows stronger, you will naturally overflow with thankfulness (Colossians 2:7). Out of sincere thankfulness will flow a compelling desire to obey Him. Regardless of the season, you will prosper (Psalm 1:1-3). With His Word rooted firmly in your heart, you can go right on producing delicious fruit and reap a huge harvest of blessing, in spite of your circumstances (Luke 8:15). You may have to drive through the salty flats once in awhile, but you sure won't have to live there.

Father, you are my hope and confidence. Thank you for faithfully carrying me from one trial to the next. Give me a faith so deep that it will never be moved by my circumstances. Amen.

64

WAKE UP!

This is why it is said: "Wake up, sleeper, rise from the dead, and Christ will shine on you." — Ephesians 5:14 (NIV)

My two-year old grandson is a morning person. Regardless of the time he goes to bed at night, he's awake by 7:00 am, and sometimes earlier. And when he's awake, he expects everyone else to be awake too. "Daddy wake up! Mama wake up!," he shouts from his bed. He's eager to greet the light of day and he doesn't want his parents to miss one minute of it. He scoots out of bed, wide awake, and filled with joy and anticipation of what the new day will bring. His parents love his exuberant personality and his zest for life. Sometimes however, they would love to catch just a few more minutes of sleep!

Sleep is a good thing. Not only do we need it to restore and replenish our bodies to stay alive and healthy, but many of us enjoy those relaxing days when we can sleep in and catch up on some much needed rest. In a state of sleep, we can detach from the world. We are unconscious of our surroundings and unaware of both the beauty and evil around us. We usually can't hear the voices of our loved ones (unless it's one of our children!). We are not aware of potential danger, and we can completely forget our problems and current situations.

The nature of sleep sounds a lot like our sinful human nature before Jesus came to shine light into our darkness. Before Jesus, we were in a deep slumber, unconscious of our surroundings and unaware of the glory and beauty of Heaven. We were unaware that we were in spiritual danger. We didn't hear the voice of God or know His faithful guidance in our daily lives.

For me, cancer was a dark bald place, but the light of Jesus broke forth into sin's darkness. During treatment, chemo and doctoring consumed most of my life, and fear and uncertainty threatened to steal my future. Perhaps, like me, your physical and emotional survival through cancer depended on clinging to the light to make it through each day. Then slowly, post treatment, life starts to normalize. Each check up confirms the absence of cancer, and every day, we walk in greater certainty that our health has returned. Praise God! However, if we're not careful, the light that shined into the darkness of our cancer crisis can start growing dim. We can easily fall into a spiritual slumber.

Jesus said, "During the day people can walk safely. They can see because they have the light of this world. But at night there is danger of stumbling because they have no light" (John 11:9-10). There are many ways we can slip back into darkness. Sometimes, our sinful nature draws us back because of lack of knowledge. We don't know the Word of God, or the Word we receive doesn't take root or is crowded out by the cares of this life (Luke 9:12-14). Sometimes we follow our sinful nature and knowingly disobey. Or, the enemy might use other people to draw us away from the light.

But there is good news for those who fall asleep! Even though your old sinful nature and your new life in Christ are in constant conflict with each other (Galatians 5:17), you are under no obligation to follow your sinful nature back into the darkness (Romans 8:12). If you confess your sins to Him, He is faithful and just to forgive and cleanse you from every wrong (1 John 1:9). He will create a clean heart and an obedient spirit within you, filled with joy and anticipation of what the new day will bring. Wake up! Rise from your spiritual slumber and Christ will shine on you!

Father, thank you that your tender mercies start fresh every day. Wake me up from this spiritual slumber and draw me back into the light! Amen.

65

COME THIRSTY

Anyone who is thirsty may come to me! — John 7:37

A few weeks ago, on a really stressful day, my tank ran empty. My to-do list was a mile long, but I ran into a brick wall with every project I tried to complete. My wheels were spinning all day long, but at the end of the day, I had nothing to show for it. With each brick wall, the frustration mounted. I could see it in my short and irritable responses to my husband, my lack of patience driving in the car, my annoyance with the slow clerk at the store, and the banker who didn't know how to help me with a simple transaction. By the end of the day, I was in full blown melt down mode. My peace was gone. A few days of operating on my own power finally caught up with me. I needed time with God, time in His presence to be refreshed, restored, and refilled with His Spirit. But the chasm that separated me from my only source of spiritual refreshment spanned as far as the eye could see. I understand how King David felt when he said: "O God, you are my God; I earnestly search for you. My soul thirsts for you; my whole body longs for you in this parched and weary land where there is no water" (Psalm 63:1).

I knew better than to allow myself into this empty state, to go and go until I literally "ran out of gas." To paraphrase the words of

David, I have seen Him in His sanctuary and gazed upon His power and glory. He rescued me from the darkest time of my life. He met me in the pit of cancer and pulled me out. I grew to understand that His unfailing love is better than life itself. I lifted my hands to Him in prayer and I know, no matter how much satisfaction I get by checking off items on my to-do list, only He can truly satisfy. I have praised Him with songs of joy (Psalm 63:2-5).

How did I get here? Jesus knew we would sometimes lose our way. He said when we grow weary of carrying the heavy burdens in this life, we could come to Him and He would give us rest for our souls. We can take His yoke instead. His yoke is easy to bear and the burden He gives us is light (Matthew 11:28-30). A yoke is a heaving wooden harness that fits over shoulders of oxen and attaches to piece of equipment that the oxen pull. In the same way, we can carry burdens of sin, the excessive demands of others, oppression for our beliefs, or simply weariness from being separated from God. The burden I carried that day resulted in a thirst that could only be quenched by spending time in His presence. In that place of rest, He promises love, healing, and peace. My to-do list may still be there, but my intimate relationship with Him changes those wearisome, overwhelming tasks into spiritual productivity and purpose.

I lay awake that night praying, soaking, and meditating on Him throughout the night. I sang for joy in the shadow of His wings, clinging to Him and knowing that, in spite of my failures the day before, His strong right hand held me securely (Psalm 63:6-8). The next morning I awoke filled and satisfied. The burden had lifted because I no longer carried it alone.

When you are running on spiritual empty, Jesus urges you to

come to Him and drink. The living water He gives you is not only the gift of eternal life, but the Holy Spirit who empowers, restores, and refreshes. He will satisfy your thirsty soul so you can receive and pour out His life giving blessings on all who come into your path. You simply can't walk in the fullness of life God intended when your soul is trapped in a parched and weary land where there is no water. You can't serve Him on an empty tank. Come for a Holy Spirit refill as often as you need. Come as often as you like. Come thirsty.

Father, thank you for carrying my burdens. Forgive me when I lose my way. Only you can truly satisfy my thirsty soul. Refresh me, Lord! Amen.

66

LONE RANGER

And let us not neglect our meeting together, as some people do,
but encourage one another, especially now that the day of his return
is drawing near. — Hebrews 10:25

Some of us believers are isolated from other Christians. It can be intentional or unavoidable, depending on our circumstances. I remember the years leading up to my diagnosis of cancer in 1999. As a private person, I thought my immediate and extended family, a couple of close friends, and some surface level acquaintances with neighbors were enough people in my life. Even though I went to church every Sunday, I wasn't engaged beyond a cordial "hello" with anyone in my large suburban mega-church. This is not so unusual. I know many Christians who have no church home at all. After my treatment ended and my life changed course, I learned what I had been missing.

God never intended for us to be isolated Christians. When we became believers, we were called into a wonderful friendship with God through His Son (1 Corinthians 1:9). The Bible makes it clear that our fellowship with Him goes two ways. In addition to vertical alignment with Him, our relationship requires horizontal alignment with others. We enter into fellowship with other

Christians (I John 1:3). It is not possible to love and live in a right relationship with God without loving and caring for other believers (1 John 2:9-10). This was evidenced in the New Testament where everyone participated in a local assembly. There was no record of Christians practicing their faith in isolation. Wherever Christians were within range of each other, they met. Every time the Apostle Paul came into a town and won a few converts, he immediately organized them into a church. For Christians in the early church, regular gathering for fellowship and preaching was a part of life (Acts 20:7).

After I began fully participating in my own local church, I learned that an isolated Christian misses out on many spiritual blessings God intended for His children. He gave us spiritual gifts, including gifts of wisdom, knowledge, faith, healing, miracles, prophesy, and discernment (1 Corinthians 12:4-10). He didn't provide these gifts for our own purposes, but so we could care for each other (1 Corinthians 12:7; I Peter 4:10). He intends for us to meet the needs of other Christians by using our strengths to help in their areas of weakness. In times of sadness, we are to comfort one another (I Thessalonians 4:18). In times of discouragement, we are to build each other up (I Thessalonians 5:11). We are to confess our sins to one another and pray for one another (James 5:16). We can't obey these Biblical directives apart from other believers.

God designed in His church to be a place where spiritual leaders could watch out for our welfare (I Peter 5:1-4; Hebrews 13:17). When we don't submit to their spiritual oversight or give anyone permission to hold us accountable in our Christian walk, we can easily rationalize sinful attitudes or actions. I have been a part of various small groups of believers for several years now and have had many situations where they have called me out on "my stuff," helped me get back on track, and prayed for me.

Your journey after cancer will be enhanced by fellowship with people who will agree in with in prayer that your healing is complete, encourage you with the promises of His word, and pray with you in times of fear. God is in the midst of our prayers when two or more are gathered and His favor and strength are multiplied in the combined faith of His people (Matthew 18:20). He honors a gathering in His name by coming into its midst with His power and anointing and often manifests spiritual gifts such as healing.

The enemy may go around like a roaring lion looking for some victim to devour and a person standing alone can be attacked and defeated; but there is strength in numbers (1 Peter 5:8; Ecclesiastes 5:12)! Paul warns the church to put on spiritual armor for protection in order to stand firm (Ephesians 6:10-18). It is essential to take every opportunity available to receive ministry from the body and strength from his Word. Please don't miss out on the blessing of Christian community. God never intended for you to be a lone ranger.

Father, thank you for providing Christian community to encourage me in my faith journey. Help me to find opportunities for authentic fellowship with other believers. Amen.

67

Walking Dead

*"What sorrow awaits you teachers of religious law and
you Pharisees. Hypocrites! For you are like whitewashed tombs —
beautiful on the outside but filled on the inside with dead people's
bones and all sorts of impurity. Outwardly you look like righteous
people, but inwardly your hearts are filled with hypocrisy
and lawlessness."* — Matthew 23:27-28

A friend of mine grew up in a small Midwestern Scandinavian community in a church that was established in the mid-1800s. The church was socially conservative at its roots and people were held to a high standard of moral character and behavior. Dancing, drinking, playing cards, and other decadent behaviors were not allowed. People caught breaking the rules or entangled in sin were held accountable by the pastor and elders of the church. My friend tells of the blatant inconsistencies he began to notice by the time he reached middle school age. Many of the same young men who were so respectful and reverent in church would go over to the local coffee shop after the service. They would scoff at the message, express doubt and cynicism over the teachings of the church, and share stories of parties, dancing, and infidelity. All this conversation was laced with curse words and enjoyed over a smoke or two before they all headed back to church for Sunday school.

Jesus called the Pharisees "hypocrites" and "whitewashed tombs" because they outwardly appeared holy, but inwardly, they remained filled with corruption and greed. They didn't obey the rules to honor God, but to make themselves look good. They knew the Scriptures, but didn't live by them. Looking holy in order to receive admiration and praise was more important to them than actually *being* holy (Matthew 23:5-7). They were so caught up in the laws and their own made up rules that they missed where the laws were pointing. As a result, they were beautiful on the outside but dead on the inside.

My friend's experience is good example of how we can have religion with no Jesus. We can know the Bible, but it doesn't change our lives. We can say we follow Jesus, but not live by His standards of love. There was a lot of Bible teaching and emphasis on head knowledge in his church, but the head knowledge didn't translate into daily life. For many, there was no real life transformation. Being a good Christian was based on outward appearances. When the Holy Spirit doesn't drive our outward behavior, we can do a lot of good things for the wrong reasons. My friend's church was not a place where he felt comfortable bringing his brokenness and receiving God's grace and restoration through the love and acceptance of others. Love and acceptance were contingent upon looking good and following the rules.

A pastor at our church used to ask this question: "Why pretend to be a Christian when you can actually be one?" We can "play church." We can do all the right things to appear religious. We can read the Bible every day, go to Bible study, serve in the church and at the local soup kitchen, and never once connect with the only one who can make us truly holy. The Apostle Paul points us to the source of life transformation: "I pray that from his glorious, unlimited resources he will empower you with inner strength through his Spirit. Then Christ will make his home in your hearts as you trust in him. Your roots will grow down into God's love and keep you strong. And may you have the power to understand, as all God's people should, how wide, how long, how high, and how deep his love is. May you experience the love of Christ, though it is too great to understand fully. *Then* you will be made complete with all the fullness of life and power that comes from God (Ephesians 3:16-19; emphasis mine)."

When you encounter Jesus through personal experience, the Holy Spirit will motivate your actions and behaviors. Holiness flows from a life transformed from the inside out. It flows out of obedience and love that is not motivated by external appearances, rules, rewards, or the approval of others. It comes from the heart, not the head. You are no longer walking dead. You are alive.

Father, you are the only One who can make me holy. Forgive me for the times I have been religious on the outside but dead on the inside. Holy Spirit, come. Change me from the inside out. Amen.

68

Change the Atmosphere

*Because of God's tender mercy, the morning light from
heaven is about to break upon us, to give light to those who sit in
darkness and in the shadow of death, and to guide us to the
path of peace.* — Luke 1:78-79

People often comment that I have the gift of hospitality. I'm
no gourmet cook and I always go for an easy-to-prepare menu,
but I do love to create ambiance when I entertain. The candles,
lighting, and table setting have to be a perfect complement to my
stone and wood floors, earth-tone walls and rugs, and dark leather
furniture. I have been in beautiful homes with white carpet, pristine
Queen Anne furniture, and exquisitely framed artwork, and felt
underdressed. People come in my home and tell me it feels warm,
inviting, and comfortable. I tell them to keep their shoes on.

In the same way that our senses perceive a certain atmosphere
from our physical surroundings, there is an atmosphere we can
discern in our spirits. Maybe you have walked into the aftermath
of a conflict between friends or co-workers, watched a disturbing
movie, dined in a restaurant, or attended a social gathering and
felt something very "off" in the spiritual realm. You sensed chaos,
darkness, or perhaps a spiritual heaviness. When I visited Buddhist

temples in Sri Lanka, the spiritual atmosphere was so dark and oppressive I could barely breathe. In contrast, when I step into the prayer chapel at our church, the presence of Jesus is so fragrant I can almost smell it.

There is a great example of contrast in spiritual atmosphere in the first and last verses in the Book of Mark. In the beginning verses, the people in His hometown of Nazareth were deeply offended and He couldn't do any mighty miracles because of their unbelief (Mark 6:3, 5). By the end of the book, the people of Gennesaret and surrounding areas were bringing the sick to Him on mats and they were healed simply by touching the fringe of His robe (Mark 6:53-56). It was the same Jesus, but an altogether different atmosphere. In this, and countless other situations, the Lord's healing power was strongly with Jesus (Luke 5:15-17).

Jesus often withdrew into the wilderness to pray (Luke 5:16). Through His constant connection with His Father in prayer, He brought the power of Heaven to earth as He healed the sick and set the captives free. The prayers of Jesus changed the atmosphere. Then, He let Peter, John, and James in on His secret. He took them up on the Mount of Transfiguration and He gave them a taste of the heavenly realm (Mark 9:2-7). Prayer created a spiritual atmosphere that was so strong with the Lord's presence in the early church that people who simply passed by Peter's shadow were healed (Acts 5: 15-16).

The entire spiritual atmosphere changed when Jesus came into the world. He was the light that broke forth from Heaven to shine into the darkness. It's no secret that the enemy is not happy with the drastic change in the atmosphere. His goal is to keep us in bondage to the power of darkness. Some people love the darkness more than the light and are content with this arrangement (John 3:18-20). As believers, we are in constant warfare against the powers of darkness, but God has not left us to our own resources. We have the power to change the spiritual atmosphere in our own realm of influence. We have the spiritual armor of God to help us stand firm against the mighty powers of darkness who rule this world (Ephesians 6:11-12). Darkness can never extinguish the light of Jesus (John 1:5). When we are filled with the Holy Spirit, our very presence brings light to the dark places.

The Prophetess Anna prayed her entire lifetime to prepare the atmosphere for the coming Messiah (Luke 2:36-38). You, too, can pray every day for the Holy Spirit to hover over your home and loved ones, for God to send His angels into your midst, and to fill your home and workplace with His presence. You can fill your house and car with Christian music and listen to it via iPod at work, at the gym, or in bed at night. Most of the words are Scripture and will bring the Word of God into your surroundings. Let Jesus change your atmosphere into a place of healing for all who enter.

Father, thank you for giving me the power through the Holy Spirit to change the atmosphere wherever I go. Help me to carry your light into the dark places of my world. Amen.

69

GOLIATH MOMENT

*Have mercy on me, O God, have mercy! I look to you
for protection. I will hide beneath the shadow of your wings
until the danger passes by. I cry out to God Most High, to God
who will fulfill his purpose for me.* — Psalm 57:1-2

After my treatment ended several years ago and my life changed
dramatically, I thought I knew what God wanted me to do. I felt
His anointing on me for ministry, and specifically for a certain
area of ministry. At first, everything fell into place. I felt forward
momentum, a strong confirmation of my calling, and a taste of
walking in my destiny. Then, everything seemed to come to a halt.
Every move I made toward my calling, I came against a brick wall.
There were "border bullies" at every turn. I began to feel like King
David with my one "Goliath moment" and then relegated to the
caves for thirteen years. In some areas of my ministry calling, I'm
still hiding in the caves!

David was anointed King of Israel but he had to wait for years
to realize God's promise. The calling itself was unmistakable. When
God sent the Prophet Samuel to Jesse's house to anoint his son
king, the Lord rejected the first seven sons Jesse presented. Finally,
Samuel ordered the youngest son, David, to come in from the field

where he was tending the sheep. Samuel knew immediately this was God's chosen one. He poured olive oil on his head and anointed him king on the spot and the "Lord came upon him from that day on" (1 Samuel 16:13).

Soon after, David had his moment of glory. When the Philistine and Israelite armies faced each other for battle, Goliath, the Philistine giant, challenged the Israelites to settle their dispute with a single combat. David, armed only with his shepherd's staff, his sling, and five smooth stones, faced Goliath's taunting threats: "You come to me with sword, spear, and javelin, but I come to you in the name of the Lord of Heaven's Armies — the God of the armies of Israel, whom you have defied. Today the Lord will conquer you, and I will kill you and cut off your head. And then I will give the dead bodies of your men to the birds and wild animals, and the whole world will know that there is a God in Israel! And everyone assembled here will know that the Lord rescues his people, but not with sword and spear. This is the Lord's battle, and he will give you to us" (1 Samuel 17:45-47)! And the Lord did. With a single stone from his sling, David toppled the giant and then killed him with his own sword.

After his triumph over Goliath, David must have had no doubt his anointing was for real. Then everything came to a halt. Saul, the current king of Israel, had deliberately disobeyed and lost favor with God. When Saul realized David would become the next king, he became jealous and obsessed with killing David. David spent the next 13 years running for his life. He wrote many of the Psalms during this time of hiding in caves and waiting for God to act. When we read his raw emotions as cries out to God for mercy, there is no doubt he wondered whether God's calling on his life would ever come to pass (Psalm 142). Yet he always ends each Psalm praising God and trusting Him to fulfill His promises.

Perhaps like David, you find yourself hiding in the caves, waiting for God to make good on His promises. He may be using this time to refine, teach, and prepare you as He prepared David for his future responsibilities as king. Saul, his predecessor, had great promise but failed due to character issues. Perhaps he wasn't ready to be king. God was getting David ready. David had many opportunities to kill Saul and speed up God's timetable, but he resisted. Don't be impatient and strive to make to make things happen. God may be using your time in the cave to build your character and get you ready. When you are tempted to doubt your calling, stand on your Goliath moment and trust God to fulfill His purpose for your life.

Father, thank you for preparing me to fulfill my destiny. Help me to trust you to make good on your promises, regardless of how long it takes. Amen.

70

Nobody Knows But Jesus

O LORD you have examined my heart and know everything about me. You know when I sit down or stand up. You know my thoughts even when I'm far away. — Psalm 139:1-2

By the time I reached the end of my journey through cancer, I had a profound revelation. No one close to me, not even my husband and children, truly understood the emotional trial I had been through. I came to the same revelation in the early years of my ministry for people with cancer. I always felt like God rescued me from the fire and then threw me back in. The natural human tendency would be to stay as far away as possible from any reminders of the emotional turmoil God had delivered me from. Instead, I found myself praying for people with a recent diagnosis, ministering to them through treatment decisions, surgery, chemo, and side effects, visiting them in hospitals, and sometimes, praying and reading Scripture at their bedside when they went home to Jesus.

I tried to explain to those close to me how difficult it was to be obedient to God's call when everything inside of me wanted to run the other direction. They usually answered with a blank stare and sometimes a comment like, "Why do it, then?" No one really understood. As the years passed, God's grace carried me through emotional challenges of surviving cancer. In retrospect, it feels as though people understand the concept of surviving cancer much better than they understand what it's like to survive as a survivor. If you have a deep need to be emotionally authentic and to be understood by people, you can join me right now in a chorus of "Nobody Knows the Trouble I've Seen."

If you're like me, you might have discovered it's not only the emotional baggage of cancer that your friends and loved ones don't understand. It may be difficult for spouses, children, parents, family and best friends to truly relate to any of your deepest emotional battles. We put a lot of pressure on those we love to meet our expectations and standards, when as human beings, we often fall short and disappoint each other. The only answer to our deep desire to be understood lies in the second line of the refrain of "Nobody Knows the Trouble I've Seen." Nobody knows but Jesus.

My husband loves me, but he can't peer into the deepest secret places of my heart. He doesn't know every single intimate thought or the source of every feeling. He doesn't know all my emotional struggles or the hidden fears, wounds, and defenses buried beyond reach of even my own understanding. Only Jesus knows. He knows everything about me. He knows when I sit down or stand up. He knows every thought before I think it. He knows what I'm going to say even before I say it (Psalm 139:4). He knows everything about me, even down to the number of hairs I lost that grew back on my head (Matthew 10:30).

When you feel as though no one truly understands, remember you have a great High Priest who knows everything about you and advocates for you before the Father in Heaven (Hebrews 4:14-15).

Jesus didn't abandon you here on earth with your own resources to cope with your troubles. Even when you can't name your feelings and you haven't a clue how to pray and what words to use, the Holy Spirit inside of you knows exactly what to pray for and how to pray. "But the Holy Spirit prays for us with groaning that cannot be expressed in words. And the Father who knows all hearts knows what the Spirit is saying, for the Spirit pleads for us believers in harmony with God's own will" (Romans 8:26-27). Nobody truly knows your hidden secrets, thoughts, fears, and yearnings. Nobody knows but Jesus.

Father, thank you for understanding those secret parts of me that my friends and family will never truly know. Help me to expect less from them and more from you. Amen.

71

Just Be

Sin is no longer your master, for you no longer live under the requirements of the law. Instead, you live under the freedom of God's grace. — Romans 6:14

My daughter was a rule follower. She had straight A's throughout her entire grade school and high school tenure. As a child, she rarely disobeyed. Unlike her older brother, I have very little recollection of having to discipline her. In high school and later in college, she stood on the sidelines while her classmates were drinking, having sex, and getting into trouble. She was critical of them because they didn't follow the rules. They didn't measure up to her standard of good behavior. All this striving and rule following began to unravel when she got her first B in college. The class was organic chemistry, an extremely difficult subject even for the brightest students. As she sobbed into the phone that night, we both realized she was on a treadmill of striving to measure up. She was tired of doing. Not only did she feel pressure to meet our expectations, but God's expectations too. She had to learn that God, as well as her earthly parents loved her, regardless of how well she performed or how well she followed the rules.

My daughter had to learn that she no longer lives under the

law, but under grace. Today, she works as a youth leader for a mega-church and carries both operational and spiritual responsibility for over 1500 students and 300 volunteer leaders. If she's not careful, she can easily jump back on the treadmill of performance and become obsessed with striving and doing to achieve perfection. She knows when she is tempted to go there, she has to stop and trust His grace to cover any mistakes or forgotten details. When she relies on His strength, she can do less and accomplish more (John 15:5). She can be the child of God He created; loved without condition.

Laws and rules define good and evil, command that we do good, judge our actions for obedience to the rules, and condemn us when we fall short. God gave the law to Moses and Israelites to show us how desperately we needed a Savior (Romans 3:20). No matter who we are or what we have done, we are only made right with God by placing our faith in His Son (Romans 3:22). Even though we live under grace because Jesus paid the price for our mistakes, many Christians still choose to live under the law. They fear judgment and condemnation, so they do more good things to measure up. But how much is enough? The truth is, we can never do enough (Romans 3:23). Paul said no one can ever be made right with God by doing what the law commands (Romans 3:20).

Some people believe that since Jesus took our punishment, we are no longer required to follow the law. But Paul made it clear that the law is still holy, right, and good (Romans 7:12) and the Apostle John instructs us to keep God's commandments (1 John 5:3). While we are constantly battling our sinful nature and the desire to disobey the law (Galatians 5:17), Paul reminds us that we under no obligation to do what our sinful nature urges us to do (Romans

8:12). Unlike the Israelites, we have the power of the Holy Spirit inside of us to help us live righteously. Our obedience to Christ becomes natural and voluntary, not because we fear punishment from the outside, but we love Him from the inside.

Under grace, you are made right with God completely apart from your works. Nothing you do will help you earn favor or avoid punishment, because you are no longer made right with God by following the rules. His love for you is perfect and is not dependent on your performance. The problem arises when you are disappointed in yourself and unconsciously pull away from God, and then attribute His distance for displeasure. Instead of going to Him for love, you just get on the treadmill and try harder. All this time, He is waiting for you to step into His grace and let Him love you. You don't have to keep doing. Just be.

Father, thank you that there is no condemnation in Jesus. Help me to stay off the treadmill of striving to earn your love and to live under the freedom of your grace. Amen.

72

MORE THAN A CONQUEROR

Who shall separate us from the love of Christ? Shall tribulation,
or distress, or persecution, or famine, or nakedness, or peril, or sword?
Yet in all these things we are more than conquerors through
Him who loved us. — Romans 8:35, 37 (NKJV)

What does it mean to be "more than a conqueror?" I wonder if Peter thought he had conquered the physical laws of nature when he impulsively jumped out of the boat and walked on water toward the loving arms of Jesus. He didn't sink until he took his focus off the Lord and looked at the high waves around him. Terrified, he shouted "Save me, Lord!" Jesus instantly reached out his hand, grabbed him, pulled him safely into the boat, and stopped the storm (Luke 14:25-31).

Peter's experience is a good example of the tension between truth and facts. Jesus represents the truth, and the storm and the water around him represent the facts. Facts are temporal and worldly, while God's truth is eternal. We must have realistic contact with the outside world and the storms that come, but we must also know that God's Word is truth whether we experience it on this earth or not. We shouldn't deny the facts, but we shouldn't let them limit us either. In His power, we can transcend the facts like Peter did.

In this world, we can have trouble, calamity, persecution, or be hungry, cold, in danger, or be threatened with death. And yes, we can have cancer. But in the midst of all these facts, we are more than conquerors. No matter what happens, we can never be separated from His love. Suffering can never sink us. It can only draw us into the power of His love, the same power that raised Christ from the dead and conquered natural law so Peter could walk on the water. Suffering doesn't mean God has abandoned you. When Peter sank, Jesus reached out and pulled him out of the water. It is impossible for Him to abandon you and leave you to drown in all your problems. His death proved His unconquerable love. Despite your hardships, overwhelming victory is yours. His eternal truth always triumphs over the facts.

For example, it may be a fact that you had cancer. The truth is, you have been healed by His wounds (1 Peter 2:24). It may be a fact that the cancer was an aggressive type. The truth is, nothing is impossible with God (Luke 1:37) and His arm is not too short to save (Isaiah 59:1). For some, it may be a fact that for some cancers, there is no cure. The truth is, everyone who keeps on asking will be given what they ask for (Luke 11:9-11). It may be a fact that cancer can come back. The truth is, no one can oppose what God does, no one can reverse His actions (Isaiah 43:13), and affliction will not rise up a second time (Nahum 1:9). It may be a fact that for some, cancer will limit life expectancy. The truth is, He will rescue and honor you in times of trouble, and satisfy you with a long life (Psalm 91:15-16). It may be a fact that hardships will come. The truth is that God, who began the good work within you, will continue his work until it is finally finished (Philippians 1:6).

Jesus commanded that we pray for God's truth to be manifest

in the world. He has given us the Holy Spirit as a foretaste of future glory until that day when we will have our full rights as His children (Romans 8:23). In the meantime, you may see inconsistencies between the truth of His Word and the facts around you. Don't be tempted to base your understanding of God on your experience and what you see in the natural. God is good and His word is truth, regardless of the inconsistencies. You have a truth that transcends all the temporal and worldly facts. You have a truth that conquered the world and all its troubles. You have Jesus. In Him, you are more than a conqueror.

Father, thank you that I am more than a conqueror in your Son Jesus. In spite of my troubles, I can never be separated from your love. Help me to know your eternal truth. Amen.

73

Let Your Old Self Die

*My old self has been crucified with Christ. It is no longer
I who live, but Christ lives in me. So I live in this earthly body by
trusting in the Son of God, who loved me and gave himself for me.*
— Galatians 2:20

Our Christian life began when we died to our old self and
became one with Christ (Romans 6:5-11). In God's eyes, we are no
longer condemned because all of our sin died with Jesus (Colossians
2:13-15). Through our faith in Him, we are instantly made right
with God (2 Corinthians 5:14). Jesus gave His life not only to free
us and cleanse us from sin, but to make us His very own people,
totally committed to growing in Christ and doing what is right
(Titus 2:14). While our sinful nature died the moment we accepted
Christ, to grow in Christ and become like Him takes a lifetime.
Paul describes it as a long and strenuous race (1 Corinthians 9:24-
27). We must regularly crucify the selfish ambitions that keep us
from following Him (Luke 9:23-25).

Fortunately, we don't have to fight this life long battle on
our own. God gave us the Holy Spirit to continue to fight our
sinful nature (Ephesians 1:19). Paul said "throw off your old sinful
nature and your former way of life, which is corrupted by lust and

deception. Instead, let the Spirit renew your thoughts and attitudes. Put on your new nature, created to be like God — truly righteous and holy" (Ephesians 4:22-24). Our choices are never completely free of the conflict between our self and the Spirit within us. As we submit to the Holy Spirit and allow our self to die, we become more and more like Jesus (Galatians 5:17).

A good way to know how you're doing on this path toward Christ likeness is to ask yourself this question: when life squeezes me, what comes out of me? Is it anger, offense, and rage or love, patience, and self-control? If you're anything like me, it all depends! On some days, I can respond with love and patience to the most aggravating situations. On other days, I confess that I've reacted in a "less than Christ-like" manner to such things as slow traffic, a long grocery store line, a disagreement with a loved one, or a hurtful comment or decision by others. The Apostle Paul sums up our struggle with sin in Romans 7:14-25 when he refers to his own sinful nature as "rotten through and through," concludes that he is a miserable person, and thanks Jesus for setting him free.

Life certainly squeezed Jesus. He faced the ultimate injustice, but He responded with silence instead of offense. After He was arrested, they made false testimony against Him, spit on Him, and beat Him until He was unrecognizable. Yet, He never said a word in His own defense (Matthew 27:14). Life squeezed a Gentile woman when she asked Jesus to heal her daughter. He told her that He should first help the Jews because "it isn't right to take food from the children and throw it to the dogs." Instead of taking offense to being called a dog, she responded, "Even the dogs under the table are given some crumbs from the children's plates." Jesus blessed her response by instantly healing her daughter (Mark 7:24-29).

When life squeezes you, what comes out? There will be plenty of opportunities to be offended and retaliate. But Jesus told us to love our enemies and pray for those who persecute us (Matthew 5:44). Instead of taking revenge, trust God to administer justice. If your enemy is hungry, feed them and if they are thirsty, give them drink. Instead of letting evil conquer you, you can conquer evil by responding in love (Romans 12:20-21). The next time you're tempted to be offended, submit to Jesus. Let Him rise up to meet the offense on your behalf. Let a little more of your old self die.

Father, thank you for your Son who gave Himself for me and for the Holy Spirit who conquers the sin in my life. The next time I am faced with injustice, help me to respond like Jesus. Amen.

74

YET YOU ARE HOLY

Every day I call to you, my God, but you do not answer.
Every night you hear my voice, but I find no relief. Yet you are holy,
enthroned on the praises of Israel. Our ancestors trusted in you,
and you rescued them. — Psalm 22:2-4

If you catch pneumonia, the doctor will take an x-ray, treat you with an antibiotic, and call you cured when the film shows no more signs of infection. It's not that way with cancer. Treatment lasts for months, and the doctor may never say you are cured, regardless of what the films and tests show. In the months and years after the treatment ends, doctors will follow you closely. A certain percentage of people will have a recurrence and they want to make sure you're not one of them. While you might appreciate their care and vigilance, all this caution does raise some anxious thoughts and questions. *Will I ever be normal again? Will I always have this dark cloud of uncertainty hanging over me? Why did I survive and others didn't? Am I really healed? Can I get on with my life? Is it really over?* Perhaps the better question is, can I praise God regardless of the outcome?

When Daniel's friends Shadrach, Meshach, and Abednego faced a fiery death in the furnace, they chose to trust God regardless of the outcome. Over 2500 years ago, King Nebuchadnezzar conquered Judah and brought them back to Babylon as captives. When he erected a ninety-foot tall gold statue and demanded people of all races and nations bow down and worship it or be thrown into a furnace, they refused: "If we are thrown into the blazing furnace, the God whom we serve is able to save us. He will rescue us from your power, Your Majesty. But even if he doesn't, Your Majesty can be sure that we will never serve your gods or worship the gold statue you have set up" (Daniel 3:17-18). The king was so enraged that he heated the furnace seven times hotter and had them thrown into the roaring flames. But the Lord rescued them and they emerged from the fiery furnace completely untouched by the fire and heat. The possibility of not being saved did not shake their faith in what they knew to be true. They stood firmly in the ongoing tension of between God's truth and the facts surrounding them, regardless of the outcome.

On this journey of survivorship, you may be tempted to compare your outcome to the outcome of others. You may try to make sense out of the fact that some are healed, some suffer recurrences, and others pass away. Peter did the same thing. After Jesus told Peter how he would die to glorify God, he responded by asking about John: "What about him, Lord?" Jesus replied, "If I want him to remain alive until I return, what is that to you? You follow me" (John 21:18-23). Jesus told Peter that John's outcome was not his concern. The Lord advised Peter to follow Him, regardless. Sometimes, like Peter, we try to compare our lives with others, either to rationalize our own level of faithfulness and devotion or to question God's justice. But we can't pull God down to our own human understanding of justice and fairness. His ways and His thoughts are higher than ours (Isaiah 55:8-9). Whatever God does is just and fair, whether or not we understand it.

Understanding God should never be a condition of our faith in Him. Until we meet Jesus face to face, we may never understand why one person gets cancer and another doesn't; why one person gets healed and another doesn't. If understanding God is a condition of our faith in Him, then really, we have no faith at all. Do we really want to worship a God who we have all figured out, and who has no more knowledge and understanding than we do? Even Job, after losing everything and enduring great suffering, concluded it was better to know God than to know why. He chose to trust God, regardless of the outcome.

I pray that what you see and experience around you never shakes your faith in what you know to be true. I pray you can praise God regardless, because you want Him far more than anything you can receive from Him. May your love for Him never depend on receiving the outcome you desire. Regardless of the outcome, yet He is holy.

Father, forgive me if I have questioned your justice and made my understanding of you a condition of my faith. Help me to praise you, regardless of the outcome. Amen.

75

STAY FREE

So Christ has truly set us free. Now make sure that you stay free, and don't get tied up again in slavery to the law. — Galatians 5:1

Through the years, I have had the great privilege of helping some other churches start prayer ministries. The pastor and a lay leader in one smaller congregation decided to convert an office into a dedicated prayer chapel and train a few lay ministers to pray for anyone coming to the chapel before and after Sunday services. The chapel would be simply furnished with an alter, anointing oil, and a few chairs for the prayer ministers to gather around the person requesting prayer. In preparation for the launching of the ministry, the pastor began inviting anyone needing prayer to come up front after each service where he and one or two prayer ministers would lay hands on them and pray. To his surprise, some members of the congregation weren't happy with the change. They wanted their pastor back at the door to shake hands with them after the service, rather than up front praying for people in need.

Maybe I'm wrong, but I wonder if the root of their unhappiness was the desire to make sure their pastor saw them in church. This story reminds me of another. I met an older man at a book signing once who had lost his wife to cancer. My heart broke for him as he expressed

His anger at God (and me!). Through the years, they had tithed their income and volunteered many hours at their local church. It wasn't fair, he said. They were good people and "followed all the rules" and she still got sick and passed away. Now, he was left alone.

The truth is, Christ died to set us free from a long list of rules! If we try to find favor with God by tithing, serving, or even attending and being seen in church, then we must follow all the rules perfectly. When we go back to a system of making ourselves right with God by keeping the law, we have separated ourselves from Christ and fallen away from God's grace (Galatians 5:3-4). We can never earn God's love or favor through deeds or service. As survivors of cancer, we can never strive to keep our health through tithing, attending or serving in church, volunteering in the fight against cancer, or being a good person. All we can do is accept His gift of righteousness through faith (Galatians 5:5). Trying to stay right with God on a daily basis through our good deeds is the same as saying His blood isn't enough to save us. And when the cross is no longer enough, we are no longer free.

Freedom in Christ does not mean you can now live to indulge in sin or fulfill your selfish desires. It means you are free from any manmade rules, methods, or special conditions for receiving God's grace and growing in Christ. It does not mean you should never serve in your church, help people, or volunteer for good causes. It means you are free to express your faith in love (Galatians 5:6). Service and love for God and others is a natural response to receiving Christ's forgiveness and grace. You serve Him from a full and thankful heart, not from anything you might gain from your efforts. When you live this way, Christ has truly set you free. Now make sure you stay free.

Father, thank you for sending your Son to set me free from slavery to the law. Help me to stay free and to love and serve from my heart. Amen.

76

Be Bold

For God has not given us a spirit of fear, but of power and of love and of a sound mind. — 2 Timothy 1:7

People tend to hold cancer survivors in high esteem. I remember the first time I gave the keynote address at an American Cancer Society Relay for Life® event and participated in the Victory Lap. Carrying purple balloons, my family and I joined other survivors and their loved ones in a lap around a track lined with luminary bags commemorating those who had lost their battle to cancer. People clapped and cheered from the bleachers as a bagpipe band followed behind us playing "Amazing Grace." Maybe you have participated in a Susan G. Komen's Race for the Cure® and were honored with a survivor breakfast and a special survivor processional and celebration ceremony. I've been celebrated and privileged to share my story many times over the years in both Christian and secular venues.

As a survivor, you too will have many opportunities to be cheered on, congratulated, and celebrated. You may be asked to share your story at fundraising events, at your church, with small groups of friends, or you may even be called to share it with strangers. You have a wonderful testimony of God's faithfulness, but something doesn't feel right. Fear creeps in. Perhaps you are uncomfortable with all the attention or intimidated by the thought of talking about your cancer experience and your faith in public. You may be afraid of what family and friends will think if you talk about Jesus in casual conversation or secular venues, a subject that many people believe should stay in church!

Take heart, you are not alone. When the Apostle Paul assigned his young protégé Timothy to pastor the church of Ephesus, Timothy was young, timid, and reserved. He faced great opposition to his message by both believers and unbelievers alike. But Paul encouraged him to be bold. God had not given him a spirit of fear and timidity, but a spirit of power, love, and a sound mind.

Sometimes fear creeps in because life as a Christian feels too overwhelming. The demands and expectations on us are more than we can meet and we simply feel inadequate. Rather than engage, our preference is to escape and hide. But God has given us a spirit of power to face those who oppose our message and hold up under trials and challenges (Luke 24:49). In Him, we have a holy courage to speak His message boldly and triumph when we undergo persecution from others.

Often, the root of fear and timidity is a lack of love for God and people. We may be afraid of letting people get too close, or afraid of God and what He might require of us. But God has given us a spirit of love, a perfect love that casts out all fear (1 John 4:18). His love inspires courage and makes us fearless in danger. The love of Christ moves our heart to bring light into the darkness. We are compelled to share His love out of obedience to Christ, and to help others who are suffering find the same hope that saved us in our own time of need.

Finally, fear and timidity can come from a mind that lacks sound judgment, leaving us feeling helpless, confused, and intellectually inadequate. But God has given us a sound mind, well balanced and self-disciplined, under the direction of the Holy Spirit.

God Himself is cheering you around the track of life and He will not waste your triumph over cancer. He will use your testimony for His glory. When you allow people and circumstances to intimidate you, you lose your effectiveness for Him. But you are not a cowering fearful slave. You are His very own child (Romans 8:15). He gave you His Spirit to overcome fear and timidity so you can to serve Him in the ways He has called you to serve. You are complete through your union with Christ who is the ruler over every power and authority (Colossians 2:10). Walk in power and love with a sound mind. Be bold.

Father, thank you for the opportunities to tell my story and testify to your glory. Please give me boldness and courage to share your message of hope with those who need to hear. Amen.

77

He's Counting On You

A spiritual gift is given to each of us so we can help each other.
— 1 Corinthians 12:7

Sometimes I meet Christians who want no part of "organized religion." When I probe deeper I often find that at some point in their lives, they were hurt or became disillusioned with "church politics." The truth is, churches are made up of people, and at one time or another, most of us are broken people! Instead of honoring and embracing each other's gifts and talents, sometimes we do the exact opposite. We may be jealous of the gifts and abilities of others, or experience resentment by others when we use our own gifts. We may compare ourselves to others with more visible gifts and pull back because we think we have nothing to offer, or we may believe that we haven't received the recognition that we deserve for our gifts and contributions. Perhaps this has been your experience in the local church. Or maybe, after God rescued you from the ashes of cancer, you are looking for ways to serve Him and use your gifts more effectively out of a grateful heart. In either case, He's counting on you.

We have all been given different gifts by the Holy Spirit to minister to the needs of the body of believers. Many people have more than one, and one gift is not superior to another. Some of these special abilities include gifts of wisdom, knowledge, faith, healing, ability to perform miracles, prophesy, discernment, speaking in tongues, interpretation of tongues, serving, teaching, encouragement, generosity, kindness, and various kinds of leadership (1 Corinthians 12:8-10; Romans 12:6-8).

The Body of Christ is just like the human body. The human body is made of many parts, all necessary for the body to function as a whole, and all functioning under the direction of the brain. In the same way, we as Christians are to function and work together under the direction and authority of Jesus (Romans 12:4-5). Christ's Body has many parts, each part has different gifts, and each part is necessary for the body to function as a whole. The Church can't function effectively if every part has the gift of leading worship anymore than the human body can function effectively if every part were an eye or an ear. If one part is missing, the whole Church is less effective (1 Corinthians 12:14-24).

Strife and division in our local churches arise when we don't appreciate and honor each other's gifting. Paul had to correct the church in Corinth because spiritual gifts had become a source of spiritual power, causing contention and disunity. Instead of functioning more effectively, the church was divided (1 Corinthians 12:1). To use our gifts effectively, we must manage them well so God's generosity can flow through us (1 Peter 4:10). We must each know our special gifts, recognize that they came from God, and understand that our gifts are different from the gifts of others, and no more or no less important. We must not hold back our gifts, but dedicate them to God and serving others. Our gifts are never to be used for our own personal gain, to manipulate others, or serve own self interests.

If you are unsure of your spiritual gifts, talk to your pastor or complete one of the many spiritual gifts inventories available online. Remember that God gives these gifts as He pleases, and we can't acquire them on our own power. Once God has revealed your gifts to you, ask Him how you can use them to build up the Body of Christ and serve your local faith community. As you look at the diversity in gifting around you, it becomes clear why one person can't be all those things, and your gifts can't do the work of the church alone. Be grateful for those with different gifts than yours. Your strengths will balance their weaknesses, and their strengths will balance yours. Together, you make up the Body of Christ. Please don't hold anything back. He's counting on you.

Father, thank you for the diverse gifts the Holy Spirit to minister to the Body of Christ. Help me to know my gifts and to use them to serve you. Amen.

78

FRIENDLY FIRE

Those who look to him for help will be radiant with joy; no shadow of shame will darken their faces. — Psalm 34:5

"Friendly fire" is a military term referring to inadvertent firing towards one's own forces while attempting to engage the enemy, particularly when the result is injury or death. Another term for friendly fire is "fratricide," a word that originally refers to the act of a person killing their brother. Unfortunately, sometimes our experience with "organized religion" or with other Christians has felt a lot like friendly fire. Instead of receiving Christ-like love and grace in the midst of our human struggles and failings, we have encountered judgment and condemnation.

I know a young woman, let's call her Angie, who was raised in the church, but is disillusioned with Christianity. Her mother-in-law is a new ager. She is kind and caring and treats Angie with love and respect. Angie's mother attends church every Sunday and has made no secret of her disappointment with Angie's life choices. She corrects her parenting skills and housekeeping deficiencies, harps on her regularly for not going to church, and is often too busy when Angie needs help or emotional support. Who is more Christ like: Angie's mom or mother-in-law? Angie is a victim of friendly fire. In her mother's attempt to bring her back into the fold, she has pushed her further away.

Unfortunately, in a well-intentioned attempt to battle back the forces of darkness, people in the church sometimes fire a direct shot at one of their own. I know other victims of friendly fire:

• Parents of a child with leukemia who were told by some in their church that they didn't have enough faith.

• A woman whose high profile marriage ended in divorce and was shunned by some in her church instead of receiving Christian care and love.

• A young woman whose church refused to baptize her baby because he was born out of wedlock.

• A couple who was told by their leaders that they weren't tithing enough of their income to the church.

• A woman whose gifting was met with jealousy by some leaders in the church instead of being affirmed, developed, and celebrated.

Our wounds feel deeper when we are hurt by people in the church. Perhaps it's because we expect more from them. We hold them to a higher standard and we're shocked when they don't meet our expectations. Unfortunately, everyone is human and will fail you at some time or another, even those closest to you. Trusting in people, even Christians, and expecting them to meet all our needs and never make mistakes will only lead to disappointment and separate us from God (Jeremiah 17:5; Psalm 146:3-4). We can't confuse the heart and nature of Jesus with the words and deeds of people in the church or people who call themselves Christians. Unlike humans who are works in progress, Jesus demonstrated perfect love and compassion. He said anyone who has seen Him has also seen the Father (John 14:9). The only one you can trust entirely without fail is God. Only God will never leave you for forsake you (Hebrews 13:5).

When fellow Christians fall short and I am hit by friendly fire, I try to take them to the throne of God's grace instead of the throne of judgment. Judgment is God's job, not mine. My job is to choose forgiveness and extend the same love and grace He extended to me (Matthew 6:14-15). Remember, our battle is not against people, but against "evil rulers and authorities of the unseen world" (Ephesians 6:12). The best way to disarm our enemies is to "heap burning coals of shame on their heads" and to conquer evil by doing good (Romans 12:20-21). When someone takes a shot at you, choose to pray for them. When I have extended grace and prayed for those who wounded me, I have seen God come in and begin to work on their failings and change their heart and mine.

Finally, as a pastor, if you have been wounded by friendly fire, I want to apologize on behalf of the Church. I encourage you to go to God for what only God can give. No shadow of shame will ever darken your face again.

Father, forgive me for holding onto bitterness toward the failings of other brothers and sisters in Christ. I receive your grace and trust you alone to heal my wounds. Amen.

79

FROM GENERATION TO GENERATION

I remember your genuine faith, for you share the faith that first filled your grandmother Lois and your mother, Eunice. And I know that same faith continues strong in you. — 2 Timothy 1:5

My husband has fond memories of his grandmother, Adena, and her desire to hand down her strong faith to her 15 grandchildren. In the midst of a stoic Scandinavian community, Grandma Adena unabashedly talked about Jesus in regular conversation and visibly incorporated her faith into daily living. His most vivid memory was how she routinely prayed over him as little boy. Like many raised in Christian homes, my husband strayed from his faith and followed a wayward path for many years as a young adult. He credits his grandmother's strong faith and her persistent prayers for his return to the Church and his deep desire to fulfill his destiny in Christ.

Paul saw in Timothy a God-given faith, inspired by his godly heritage that would enable him to live boldly in the fulfillment of his calling in Christ. His grandmother Lois and his mother Eunice were early Christians, possibly converted through Paul's ministry in Lystra (Acts 16:1-3). They had communicated their strong and genuine faith to Timothy, even though his father was a Greek and did not share in their beliefs (Acts 16:4). To appreciate the value of a godly heritage, one only needs to contrast Timothy with King Ahaziah who was "evil in the Lord's sight" and whose mother "encouraged him to do wrong" (2 Chronicles 22:3-4). King Ahaziah was the grandson of the evil Queen Jezebel who killed off the Lord's prophets (1 Kings 18:4) and whose name is used as a synonym for evil in Revelations 2:20.

Moses gave instructions for passing on our faith heritage when he told the Israelites to repeat God's commands "again and again to your children "and to "talk about them when you are at home and when you are on the road, when you are going to bed and when you are getting up" (Deuteronomy 6:7). It was God's desire to keep his covenant and lavish His unfailing love for a thousand generations on those who obeyed His commands (Deuteronomy 7:9). Unfortunately, there is no guarantee our children will follow in our footsteps, no matter how effectively we impart our faith to them. Instead of coming to their own personal faith in Jesus, many will reject the Christian message in favor of instant gratification in a tempting and enticing world. Like the Israelites before us, our children and grandchild can lose our vision. They may have heard of His love and faithfulness, but they don't know Him. They haven't experienced Him firsthand. He is our God, not theirs.

We can take great hope in the Scripture promise that a child trained up to choose the right path will remain on it (Proverbs 22:6). We can also model our faith and pray like Grandma Adena. Your children and grandchildren have observed your triumph over cancer. You had the opportunity to model your faith in crisis and you have ongoing opportunities to model Christian character. When challenges arise in your home, you can choose to love unconditionally. You can continue to let His love, helpfulness, peace and joy shine through you, regardless of the circumstances. You can share the source of your hope in the context of daily life. You can make God part of your daily experience, not just a Sunday morning activity. Your children and grandchildren will see your faith in action when you make a habit of saying, "let's pray about that" or "we'll have to trust God for that" throughout the normal challenges of life.

Finally, pray for your children, your children's children, and the generations beyond. Pray that they will all come to know and love Jesus. Pray that the faith that sustains you, a genuine faith that may have been passed down from your own parents or grandparents, will continue to be strong in your family from generation to generation.

Father, thank you for my faith heritage and for all those who prayed for me. Help me to pass my faith on to my children and grandchildren so future generations may tell of your glory and fulfill their destiny in Christ. Amen.

80

To the Woodshed

I will not judge those who hear me but don't obey me, for I have come to save the world and not to judge it. — John 12:47

I remember the first time I fasted for an extended length of time. I had been on short fasts, skipping meals to pray about a specific issue or even day long fasts in preparation for a ministry session. This time, I went on a three week fast, abstaining from most foods and beverages to focus on spiritual growth. As in all Biblical fasting, my purpose was to deny myself something of the flesh to glorify God, enhance my spirit, and go deeper in my prayer life. I anticipated a time of deeper intimacy with Him and receiving more understanding of His plans for my life. Much of the fast turned out as I expected. For one thing, I realized how often I depended on food to satisfy me in times of restlessness instead of spending time with God. I also had several breakthroughs in my prayer life. What I didn't expect was conviction. God took me to His woodshed and revealed a specific situation where I had been holding on to bitterness and didn't trust His plans or His timing. He gently corrected me so I could receive His forgiveness and get back on track.

There is a difference between God's woodshed of conviction

and condemnation. Conviction comes from God as He gently reveals our sin. The result is a godly sorrow that leads to repentance (Romans 2:4). God holds back His judgment and patiently waits for us to come to Him so He can show us His love and compassion (Isaiah 30:18). When we do, He promises to forgive and cleanse us from every wrong (1 John 1:9). The acts of confessing to God shows that we are coming in agreement with Him that we have done wrong and are willing to turn from it. To avoid mistaking His patience and kindness for ongoing approval of our wayward ways, we can ask Him to reveal our sin. Some of us might try fasting. The conviction that results helps ensure that we don't hide our mistakes from Him or ourselves. It keeps us in the light, basking in the freedom He died to win for us. It also helps us know that as human beings, we are not perfect, but we can always be assured of His power to overcome our shortcomings.

Condemnation, on the other hand, comes directly from Satan. Whenever you hear a voice that tears you down, points out your failures, tells you how badly you messed up, and doles out punishment, you can be sure it is not the voice of God. There is no condemnation in Christ (Romans 8:1). He came to save the world, not condemn it. It is Satan who accuses the family of God (Revelations 12:10). He rubs your face in your mistakes and gives you no hope or solution for moving forward.

But there is always a solution, and God's gentle conviction will lead you there. The Blood of Jesus saves and cleanses you from every mistake you will ever make. God convicts and restores you to life. Satan punishes and condemns you to death. Conviction draws you closer to God, while condemnation keeps you away. I don't know about you, but I'll go to the woodshed with God anytime.

Father, thank you for your kind and gentle conviction when I stray from your ways. Please reveal to me when I should come to You for cleansing so I can stay in the light of your presence. Amen.

81

GOOD ENOUGH

By his divine power, God has given us everything we need for living a godly life. We have received all of this by coming to know him, the one who called us to himself by means of his marvelous glory and excellence. — 2 Peter 1:3

God is a God of excellence. He made that very clear when He gave detailed instructions to the Israelites for building the Tabernacle, exactly according to the plans He showed them (Exodus 29:5). In Exodus 25-31, He gave them a blueprint with specifications for the framework, dimensions, and materials to be used for the Tabernacle and its furnishings. He included detailed plans for the Ark of the Covenant, the table, lamp stand, alters, and the priest's clothing, right down to the tinkling bells attached to the bottom of the Aaron's robe (Exodus 25:9). When He was finished with His instructions, He assigned craftsmen and gifted them with wisdom, skill, and intelligence to complete the work (Exodus 36:1). Exodus 35-40 records the actual construction, with Moses inspecting each piece to make sure it was crafted exactly as the Lord commanded (Exodus 39:42).

God sets the bar for excellence. I want to be the best wife, mother, grandmother, author, pastor, and teacher I can be. But if I'm not careful, my desire for godly excellence can slip into perfectionism. Perfectionism is a counterfeit of excellence. It is a lie planted by Satan that tells me my best is never good enough. It leaves me anxious and worried that I might fail. It causes me to strive for the praise and approval of people instead of God. It deceives me into thinking I am solely responsible for the results of my efforts. Perfectionism causes me to live in fear and frustration, and to never be fully satisfied with my performance, and often, the performance of others.

When I live according to God's standard of excellence, I put forth my best effort and leave the rest up to Him. Instead of working for the praise and approval of people, I work only for God (Colossians 3:23). I depend on Him for results, because I know I can do nothing apart from Him (John 15:5). I live in peace knowing He is pleased with me because I'm doing my best for His glory, not mine.

Over the years, I've learned that God cares much more about perfecting me than perfecting my skills in parenting, grandparenting, writing, pastoring, or anything else I do for Him. The only way I am perfect is in Christ. By His divine power, I have everything I need to complete the work He assigns to me. I am free of the bondage of perfectionism and free from striving to measure up. His power is made perfect in my weakness (2 Corinthians 12:9). If you are struggling with perfectionism, please repent and renounce the lie that you can never be satisfied with your performance. Release the results of your efforts to God. By His marvelous glory and excellence, your best is always good enough.

Father, forgive me for striving for excellence on my own and for the wrong motives. Help me remember I am only performing for you. Amen.

82

Out of Bounds

You can make many plans, but the Lord's purposes prevail.
— Proverbs 19:21

I'm a planner. Years ago, cancer tried to steal my need to think and strategize about the future, but now I'm back in the game in full force. It's not always a good thing. Where cancer made me pause and focus on today, now I can get way out ahead of myself. My thinking and planning can take me places God is not ready for me to go. I'm naturally wired this way. My top two strengths identified by the Gallup StrengthsFinder® are strategic and intellection. No wonder I'm always jumping the gun. Instead of focusing on today and not worrying about tomorrow, I'm not only solving the problems of today, but I'm trying to solve the problems I might encounter in the future. It's a shadow side of a strategic thinker. If I can plan ahead, I can anticipate the mines in the mine field in front of me and make plans not to step on them. When I go too far down this path, my husband reels me in. He tells me I'm "out of bounds."

It's a simple sports analogy. A ball hit or thrown out of bounds is out of play. The play stops, the game resets, and often some sort of penalty is applied, whether a strike, a down, or a point for the opposing team. It's the same way with my thinking. I have to stop and reset my mind before the day can resume according to God's plan. With the Holy Spirit's help, I have to set my mind on Jesus, listen for His voice, and follow His lead (John 10:27). I can't hear His voice when my mind is spinning out of control in a multitude of different directions solving problems that might never become a reality. I need to respond to His plans for my day, instead of making plans and strategies for tomorrow. He is in the present. He'll take me into the future when He's good and ready.

Of course, some planning is a necessary part of life. Planning that results in conjecture, what ifs, and worry is not. When my mind goes out of bounds, I'm really being held in bondage to the idol of control. God created me anew to do good things and to fulfill the plans He made for me long ago (Ephesians 2:10). Not my plans, but His. For me, the last frontier of rebellion to live according to His will and not mine is my mind. When I let the Holy Spirit control it, there is life and peace. When I follow my sinful nature and my own plans, there is death (Romans 8:6). By His grace and mercy, I can be free from compulsive planning if I repent my need to control every potential detail and my lack of trust in God for tomorrow. I can renounce the lie that my plans are better than His and that He can't be trusted with my future. I can receive the truth and assurance that His plans and His timing are perfect.

You can too. You can live within the boundaries of today and rejoice in it (Psalm 119:24). Don't concern yourself with tomorrow. Tomorrow will have its own problems and there are more than enough problems to cope with today (Matthew 6:34). He won't show you exactly what the future will bring, but He will equip you to avoid every land mine in the mine field you will encounter along the way. There is no problem in your future that He hasn't already anticipated and put a solution in motion. Whether or not you slip of out of bounds, the Lord's plans and purposes will always prevail.

Father, thank you for reeling me back in when my mind roams out of bounds. Help me to trust you for tomorrow and live in the joy of today. Amen.

83

So You Think You Need a King?

"Give us a king to judge us like all the other nations have."
— 1 Samuel 8:4

A few years ago, I was questioning whether or not to continue writing and how to navigate through the world of publishing. I had been toying with the idea of finding a mentor who knew the business and could lead me through some of the challenges I encountered. When I brought the idea to my small group, we prayed and they encouraged me. I came home that night, convinced that I would begin my search for a mentor or writing coach the very next day. As I was getting ready for bed, I heard a distinct voice in my spirit: "So you think you need a king?" Immediately, I dropped to my knees. Never mind, God!

God was speaking to me through a story recorded in 2 Samuel 8:1-22. When Samuel retired as judge of the Israelite nation, he appointed his sons to be judges. Unfortunately, they were not godly leaders, so the people asked Samuel for a king. Upset, he took their request to God. God told Samuel that he should give the nation their king because the people were rejecting His leadership. Samuel went back to the people and warned them of the great price they would pay for having a political system that would take away their possessions and freedoms. But they still insisted on a king to give them victory in battle instead of God who repeatedly delivered them. They rejected God and chose to run their nation by human strength. While this is a Scripture about the government of a nation, the same holds true for how we choose to operate in our personal life. If we rely on people for leadership instead of God, we will bear the consequences (Psalm 146:3). The Prophet Jeremiah warned: "Cursed are those who put their trust in mere humans, who rely on human strength and turn their hearts away from the Lord" (Jeremiah 17:5).

The Israelites' basic problem was disobedience. If they had fully surrendered to God's leadership, they would have thrived (Deuteronomy 28:1). Paul said if we surrender ourselves to God and let Him transform us by changing the way we think, then we will know His perfect will (Romans 12:1-2). Often, instead of fully surrendering to God and seeking His will and counsel, we take the more convenient route. We pick up the phone and consult with a friend. Or we might find a mentor or coach to lead us through life's challenges.

God always gives us wisdom when we ask in faith (James 1:5-6). Sometimes, He allows others to participate in the process of imparting wisdom. There is nothing wrong with seeking the counsel of people. There are many verses in the Bible that encourage us to do so (Proverbs 11:14; 12:15; 15:22; 20:18; 24:6). David listened to Abigail and Moses listened to Jethro. David should have listened to Joab. But there should always be a balance between seeking and listening to God and listening to the counsel of man. We should always go to God first. We can trust that He has given us a sound mind to make decisions (2 Timothy 1:7). Through the Holy Spirit within us, we can begin to know God's thoughts, talk to Him in prayer, and expect Him to answer. Through Him, we have the mind of Christ (2 Corinthians 2:15-16).

In the season I was in, God wanted me to sit at His feet, not at the feet of an earthly king. When God leads you to seek the counsel of man, make sure the person is filled with goodness and able to speak truth (Romans 15:14). He or she must be knowledgeable of the Bible and able to discern good from evil (Hebrews 5:13-14). Never seek the counsel of the ungodly (Psalm 1:1-3), never view godly counsel as the final authority, and always test it to make sure it lines up with God's Word (1 John 4:1-2). When a decision is required, act with the best revelation you have. Sometimes, you may have to move forward with no clear confirmation from God, and trust that doors will close or there will be a persistent uneasiness in your spirit if you are moving outside of God's plan. If He doesn't stop you, don't doubt yourself. Remember, God knows the desires of your heart. When your heart is fully aligned with His, you don't need an earthly king. You have direct access to the King of all Kings.

Father, thank you that you are my King and I can always come to you for divine wisdom. Help me to always discern your truth in the counsel I receive from others. Amen.

84

Pray in Confidence

Now this is the confidence that we have in Him, that if we ask anything according to His will, He hears us. And if we know that He hears us, whatever we ask, we know that we have the petitions that we have asked of Him. — 1 John 5:14-15 (NKJV)

"Lord, if it be your will, please do such and such...." As a pastor of prayer, I often hear this caveat placed in front of someone's prayer request. I understand that we often do this out of reverence to God and His sovereign will, and sometimes, it's appropriate to do so. But when we add "if it be your will, Lord" to every petition we make of God, there is no need for us to stand in faith that we will receive what we ask for. Essentially, we are preparing ourselves in advance for Him to say "no." When He doesn't answer, we conclude that our prayer was outside of His will. In reality, we didn't pray in confidence according *to* His will.

When we know God's will, we can pray specifically and without doubt. Scripture tells us that we can be confident He hears us when we ask according to His will, and since He hears us, we can also be confident He will give us what He ask for. So how do we know God's will so we can pray in accordance with it? The best place to start is Scripture. When we pray the truth of Scripture over our situation, we can be confident and expectant, knowing He will answer. Sometimes, I hear a cancer survivor pray, "If it's your will, Lord, keep me well." What they are really praying, is "Lord, if it's *not* your will to keep me well, then let this cancer come back and take me!" That doesn't sound like Jesus to me, nor does it align with the mandate He left with His disciples to "lay hands on the sick and heal them" (Mark 16:18)! Jesus died to save, heal, and deliver you so you can thank God for your wellness without adding an "if it be your will." You can bring all your practical needs to God and pray in confidence that He will supply from His glorious riches (Philippians 4:19).

In addition to knowledge of the Scriptures, you can know the will of God by simply resting in His presence. Psalm 46:10 invites you to "be still and know that I am God." In your quiet times with Him, He might highlight a specific Scripture to reveal His will to you, or you may have a dream or vision, or hear a still small voice in your spirit. Occasionally, you might receive a prophetic word from a trusted source. Paul gives us deeper insight in knowing God's will when he urges total surrender: "I plead with you to give your bodies to God because of all he has done for you. Let them be a living and holy sacrifice — the kind he will find acceptable. This is truly the way to worship him. Don't copy the behavior and customs of this world, but let God transform you into a new person by changing the way you think. Then you will learn to know God's will for you, which is good and pleasing and perfect" (Romans 12:1-2).

Even when we don't know God's will, we can pray in faith because the Holy Spirit knows the will of Father God and prays for us in harmony with God's will (Romans 8:27). Jesus is interceding for us at God's right hand (Romans 8:34). What a comfort to know that the Holy Spirit seeks the depths of our hearts and prays with and for us, even when our thoughts and desires may yet be without form! Through the Spirit, the prayers of Jesus become ours and ours become His. Instead of coming to God with my laundry list of petitions and praying "if it be your will," I can know my prayers will align with His and pray in confidence!

When you pray, enter His courts with thanksgiving (Psalm 95:2). Tell God exactly what you want Him to do. Remember, Jesus made the blind man Bartamaeus declare his desire to be healed (Mark 10:51)! Don't cry out for mercy without telling Him why you need it. Don't ask for forgiveness without naming the sin you need to be delivered from or pray for His blessing without naming the areas in your life that you want to be blessed. Specific prayer helps you to know whether your greatest desires align with His. It helps you to wait in faith for the things you ask and to know when your prayers are answered. When you ask according to His will, you can pray in confidence the answers will come.

Father, thank you for the promise of answered prayer. Help me discern your will so I can pray with confident expectation. Amen.

85

Surprise Me!

"For I know the plans I have for you," says the Lord. "They are plans for good and not disaster, to give you a future and a hope."
— Jeremiah 29:11

I don't like surprises. I've even been told I'm "not adaptable." That's why I panicked a few years ago when I opened my mail box and found a bulky envelope postmarked from India. Before I even opened the envelope, I was already praying, "Please God, don't make me go to India!" Inside the envelope was an invitation to come and teach at a women's conference. I had no more started this argument with God, when a pastor in my own church invited me to join a team going to India and to teach at a women's conference our church was sponsoring. I kept giving God all my excuses. I'm not a good traveler. I didn't plan this trip. The costs are prohibitive. Every time I turned around, I was barraged with literature, billboards, advertisements, and television shows, all relating to India. Finally, I got a letter in the mail from my publisher. They were pleased to inform me that first book I had written was going to be published in, you guessed it, India. I threw the letter up in the air and said, "Ok God. I get it. You win." I went and it changed my life. Now, I'm off on another adventure. As of this writing, my husband and

I are part of a team going to Japan to provide spiritual aftercare to the victims of the earthquake that occurred on March 11, 2011. It was not on my radar screen. God surprised me. I argued with Him for a few days and lost.

One of the main reasons we struggle so much with surrendering our will to God is we don't know what He's going to do or expect from us. The root of that fear is our struggle to believe God is always good and has only the best in store for us. When I hold tight to the reigns, avoid His plans, or never dare to ask God to surprise me, it comes from a belief that He's not on my side and He has plans for disaster. But if I say, "Bring it, God! Whatever you have in store for me, I'm in!," it comes from a belief that He's always on my side, He wants to give me a future and a hope, and He will always pursue me with His goodness (Psalm 23:7). It comes from a belief that His will is always good and pleasing and perfect (Romans 12:2). I'm learning that being in His perfect will in a dangerous country on the other side of the world can be safer than being outside of His will in my own living room!

Sure, I can do things for God according to my own plans. My plans will probably be more convenient and more likely to let me stay in my comfort zone. But the Scripture says, "Unless the Lord builds a house, the work of the builders is wasted. Unless the Lord protects a city, guarding it with sentries will do no good" (Psalm 127:1). We can't make the mistake of leaving God out of our plans, just because we're afraid of where He might take us. If we do, our accomplishments will be futile.

When you trust God with the details of your future, you may never be certain where the path may lead, but you can always be certain of God and His goodness. Are you ready for new plans, new opportunities, and new adventures that stretch you, make you trust Him more, draw you closer to His heart, and make you more like Him? Go ahead and tell Him. "Bring it, Lord! Surprise me!"

Father, thank you that your plans for me are always good and pleasing and perfect. Help me to trust you when you call me out of my comfort zone. Amen.

86

THE REAL DEAL

Dear children, let's not merely say that we love each other;
let us show the truth by our actions. — 1 John 3:18

My husband is an extrovert with a successful lifelong career in sales and marketing. He's an action guy who loves Jesus. Need I say more? I've seen Him express God's love by praying with strangers at gas stations while on motorcycle trips, sharing His faith with the person sitting next to him on an airplane, and bagging groceries for people while waiting in a long line at the grocery store. It's second nature to him. A few weeks ago, we were on prayer team and the people were invited up to the front after the service if they needed us to pray for them. Long after the crowds thinned out, he noticed a couple way in the back who seemed to be struggling, but didn't come forward. This is no small sanctuary. It seats 2500 people. He went back to them and asked if everything was okay, and spent quite awhile praying for them. The next day, the husband of the couple was at our kitchen table, and later that week, he was the newest member of my husband's small group. My husband is the real deal.

Real love is action. It is the sacrificial giving of self, time, finances, or possessions in a way that helps others without expecting anything in return. Real love is a choice not a feeling. It isn't the lustful, feel good, "all about me" love that is so prevalent in our culture today. It is a decision to act in love, based solely on our love for Christ, because He loved us first (1 John 4:19). He is the source of all love, and showed His love was real by His actions. He sacrificed His life so we might have life through Him (1 John 4:9-10). It has been said that they didn't need nails to hold Him to the cross. His love would have held Him there. His love is outward, not inward. It is selfless, not selfish. To love like Jesus requires us to put our own wants and needs aside, and put the needs of others first.

The Apostle John said, "since God loved us that much, we surely ought to love each other" and "if we love each other, God lives in us, and his love is brought to full expression in us" (1 John 4:11-12). When we think about acting in a love that fully expresses God, we can begin to feel guilty. I'm nothing like my husband. I'm more reserved and introspective. I've learned over the years that God isn't telling me to go out and love more people, but to love the people He has given me to love. He expects me to love my family, my close friends, my readers, and the people He brings to me in ministry with a love that expresses His love.

If you are feeling like you don't love enough, set your heart on God's love. He knows both the motives of your heart as well as your actions, and He cares more about your true motives. When your actions fall short, the accusing voice of guilt does not come from God, because there is no condemnation in Him (Romans 8:1). God is much greater than our conscience and shortcomings (1 John 4:20).

Likewise, you can do a lot of things for God with the wrong

heart. Love is more important than how you use your gifts to serve Him (1 Corinthians 13:3). Great acts of faith and sacrifice for others have little effect without love. It's all about the heart. Real love can only come through the power of the Holy Spirit within us.

Who is God calling you to love? If you are like my husband, maybe you'll be seeking out strangers with cancer in clinic waiting rooms to offer prayer or an encouraging word. Perhaps your gifts are more practical and you'll show your love to those battling cancer by bringing meals, caring for their children, providing transportation, or sitting with them during their chemo sessions. Pray that God will break your heart for the things that break His. Pray that you can love like he loves, and show the truth by your actions. Be the real deal.

Father, thank you for loving me first and for demonstrating your love by your actions. Through the power of the Holy Spirit, help me to love like you love. Amen.

87

NOT OF THIS WORLD

I'm not asking you to take them out of the world, but to keep them safe from the evil one. They do not belong to this world any more than I do. Make them holy by your truth; teach them your word, which is truth. Just as you sent me into the world, I am sending them into the world. — John 17:15-18

Sooner or later, it happens to everyone who makes a decision to follow Jesus. We go to a family gathering, travel with colleagues for business, or gather with old friends. Conflict arises where perhaps there was no conflict before. We might be bothered by the language, the conversation, the activities, or the jokes. We say grace before a meal, where they say "bon appetite." We see hope and healing, where they see a world of limitations. We see a God who is still on the throne, where they see a hopelessly broken political system. Different morals, values, goals, and truths are driving us now. Our commitment to follow Jesus can separate us from friends and loved ones who don't make the same commitment. How do we maintain loving relationships with them? Should we? What does it actually look like to live *in* the world but not be *of* the world?

The world is an evil place. I would challenge anyone who doesn't believe in Satan to pick up the newspaper or turn on the nightly news. Take a look at the advertisements, the movies at your local theater, the Internet, and the lineup on prime time TV. To protect ourselves and our loved ones from the violence and moral decay surrounding us, we might be tempted to completely separate from the world. We only maintain Christian friendships, home school our children, or send them to Christian schools. We put locks on our TVs and computers, only watch Christian movies and television, listen to Christian radio, read Christian books, and follow Christian news networks. Our entire social life centers on our faith communities. Don't get me wrong. None of these things are wrong in and of themselves. But if we're not careful, we will find ourselves living in a Christian bubble, completely isolated from the world around us. Our old friends and family members think we're "a little strange," or worse, that we "joined a cult." The Barna Research Group found that most young Americans believe Christians are judgmental, anti-homosexual, hypocritical, too political, and sheltered. Ouch.

Jesus warned that we would risk the disapproval of those closest to us to gain a relationship with Him. When we "pick up our cross" and publicly identify with Him, we will experience opposition (Matthew 10:38-39). Families can split when some choose to follow Him and others don't (Luke 12:53). But He is not necessarily encouraging isolation or conflict. He didn't ask God to take us out of the world. On the contrary, He sent us into the world to be salt and light and to do the work He called us to do (Matthew 5:13-16). He asked the Father to protect us from evil. It's very difficult to be salt and light if we live in a bubble and don't have any relationships with non-believers in the outside world.

Jesus didn't separate Himself from the sinners. Instead, he hung out with them (Mark 2:15-17). He didn't engage in their sinful behavior, but He built relationships with them, loved them, and led them to repentance. Just as God sent His Son into the world, His Son sent you to engage in the world around you. The non-believers in your path are not "projects" you choose to befriend so you can bring them into the fold. You love them because Jesus loves them, and you probably like them too! As you invest in relationships with non-believing friends and loved ones, people are watching you. They know you are a Christ follower. They may be waiting for you to show your "true colors" and validate their opinion of Christians. You don't necessarily participate in all of their behaviors or activities, but you don't make them feel guilty either. You don't judge them. Instead, you love them. If they are hurting or need help, you don't avoid them. Instead, you show compassion and offer to pray. If they hurt you, you don't take offense. Instead, you show grace. They come to trust you. They know your values and convictions, but they have experienced a genuine, Christ-like love. They want what you have. They start asking questions about this Jesus and what a life in Him is all about.

Wherever He sends you, you carry His presence in your heart. You are breaking into the darkness with His light and His love, whether or not you say a single word about Jesus. He sent you into the world for this purpose, and He will protect you from evil. You are not of this world.

Father, thank you for sending me into the world and protecting me from the evil one. Help me to invest in others and be the full expression of your love in all of my relationships. Amen.

88

Lost in His Glory

Let all that I am praise the LORD; with my whole heart,
I will praise his holy name. — Psalm 103:1

Our church of over 6500 attendees is blessed by a 2500 seat worship center and a worship and tech team who were born to make music for the King. Week in and week out, their job is to usher the Body of Christ into the very presence of God through anointed praise and worship music. For me, it's very difficult to worship the Creator of the entire universe without being completely overwhelmed by the significance of who He really is. This is the same God who held the oceans in His hand, who measured off the heavens with His fingers, and picks up the islands as if they had no weight at all (Isaiah 40:12,15). He is the one who makes the clouds His chariot and rides upon the wings of the wind (Psalm 104:3), and who names the stars, brings them out one after another, and calls each by name to see that none are lost or strayed away (Isaiah 40:26). The more He reveals His power and majesty during worship, the more I realize how unworthy I am to stand in His presence without His grace. Sometimes, that knowledge moves me to tears. As the Lord soothes and refreshes me in the depths of my spirit, the tears wash my eyes clean, leaving me open and exposed before the Creator of all things. His tender mercy flows over me, and I'm lost in His glory.

Some people don't see worship this way. After the service recently, a man stormed past the welcome center and out the door, while complaining loudly about having to stand and sing for a half an hour before the message started. True worship is more than singing praise songs on Sunday morning. True worship is a matter of the heart. God reveals Himself to us through His Word and His presence, and we are free to respond in reverence, adoration, and gratitude from a contrite and humble spirit. If we open our hearts to Him, deep worship inspires us to hunger for more of God. Just worshipping in church on Sunday doesn't fill that hunger.

In essence, we can praise and worship Him every day, in everything we do. Whenever we live in a way that brings Him honor and glory, we are worshipping. The contentment, excitement, and purpose we feel when we do what we were created to do are strong statements of our worship. Prayer, reading Scripture, tithing, witnessing, serving, and living out our faith, if done out of reverence and submission to God, are all acts of worship.

To understand true worship, let's look at the first time the word "worship" appears in Bible. In Genesis 22, God told Abraham to sacrifice his son Isaac to test Abraham's capacity to obey Him. When Abraham saw the place God instructed him to go from a distance, he said to his servants: "Stay here with the donkey. The boy and I will travel a little farther. We will worship there, and then we will come right back" (Genesis 22:5). Abraham obeyed God, and responded by worshipping Him, even though he must have been troubled, confused, and heavy hearted. He knew his worship would cost him his son, his hope for the future, and his most precious possession. Yet, he was willing to give God the treasure of his heart because he loved Him. His humble response glorified God and his faith delighted God's heart. Abraham placed all that He was and all he had at the altar of obedience and submission, and trusted God for the outcome. As a result, God spared his son and made him the father of a nation.

This is the essence of true worship. We worship God for who He is, out of obedience, whether it makes sense or not. Come today with a submissive heart to praise and worship the God who gives hope. Lift your hands in holiness (Psalm 134:2), and hope in His grace, His promises, and His power. Stand in His house and shout praises to His name (2 Corinthians 20:19). Worship Him in holy fear and awe (Hebrews 12:28-29), giving honor and praise to the King of all Kings. If you can't physically stand before Him, then let your whole heart stand up before Him in full attention. Take all that you are and yield it to all that He is. Let all that is within you praise the Lord. Worship Him and get lost in His glory.

Father, thank you for revealing yourself to me through your Word and your presence. Help me respond to who you are by giving you my whole heart in praise and worship. Amen.

89

One Road

I am the way, the truth, and the life. No one can come to the Father except through me. — John 14:6

So many roads…so little time. We could tour the country on our Gold Wing motorcycle for a lifetime and never ride them all. The highways and byways of America spread out across the land, bound only by the vast oceans on both sides, spreading across mountains and plains, through farmland and deserts, and over lakes and streams. I have fond memories of driving through the lush rolling hills and river bluffs of Wisconsin, the red rock formations in the southwest desert and the aspen forests of the Colorado Rockies. I also remember a trip to the Blue Ridge Parkway when we got very lost on our way from Buckhannon, West Virginia to Maysville, Kentucky in pouring rain. We drove around for hours and ended up back where we started. All this, with a GPS on the bike. It showed us the way, but we had some trouble in the execution!

Life can be a lot like this. Sometimes, we try to navigate on our own without a map or a GPS and end up broken and lost. Sometimes, we believe we're on the right road and that Jesus has mapped the way. We forge ahead following our destiny, only to find something got lost in the execution. We're riding the road of life without His daily guidance and power. We start out with plan but we never arrive at our destination. We forgot that Jesus didn't merely show us the way. He *is* the way. He is the way, the truth, and the life.

Jesus made this profound statement to His disciples as He was preparing to leave them. He said He was the only road to the Father (John 4:3-6). Peter made the same statement when he said "there is no other name in all of heaven for people to call on to save them" (Acts 4:12). On the back of our Gold Wing, we have a license plate holder engraved with the words: *There Is Only One Road… Jesus.* In the politically correct culture today, these words can cause heads to turn. Some say believing that Jesus is the only road leading to redemption is narrow minded and elitist. They are offended that Christians think Jesus is the only pathway to God. Ironically, rather than being narrow and elitist, His way is wide enough for the entire world enter, if the world chooses to believe in Him.

Jesus showed He is the way through His life on earth, His death on the cross, and His intercession for us in Heaven. He is both God and man. By uniting our life to His, we are united with the Creator (John 15:10). When Jesus said "anyone who has seen me has seen the Father," He revealed Himself as God (John 14:7-9). He is the visible tangible image of God. His death and resurrection opened the way for us to boldly enter into the throne room of God (Hebrews 10:19-20). Jesus, our merciful and faithful High Priest, lives forever to plead with God on our behalf (Hebrews 2:17-18; 7:24-25).

Jesus showed He is the truth, because He is the reality of all God's promises. His sacrifice on the cross was the embodiment of God's love. Jesus didn't just teach the truth, He is the truth. He is the source of all truth, the truth that sets us free from the bondage of sin, and the perfect standard for what is true and right (John 8:32). As we seek Him and live in obedience to His teachings, His perfect truth frees us to be all that God calls us to be.

Jesus is the life, because He joins His divine life to ours, now and forever. Through His redemptive work, we were reconciled to the Father and born into a new life in the Spirit (Titus 3:5). Jesus offers a life in all its fullness (John 10:10), a peace the world cannot give (John 16:33), a love that surpasses human knowledge (Ephesians 3:19), and a life overflowing with joy (John 15:11).

Jesus didn't just leave you here on earth without a map. He doesn't show the way, and leave the execution up to you and your faulty GPS. You have the living Christ dwelling inside of you to guide you, teach you, and bless you abundantly. He is the way to know and experience God as your heavenly Father, and the very road you travel. He is the truth, your standard for living, and the very truth that sets you free. He is your assurance of eternal life, and the very life you long to live today. He is the way, the truth, and the life. There is only one road.

Father, thank you for providing a sure road that leads to you. Help me to walk in your ways, live in your truth, and dwell in your abundant life today and forever. Amen.

90

Better Than the Old

This means that anyone who belongs to Christ has become a new person. The old life is gone; a new life has begun!
— 2 Corinthians 5:17

In the beginning of this book, a reader named Carla vividly described the "new normal" that many experience in the aftermath of cancer. She found herself living in a holding pattern, waiting for proof that the crisis is truly over and she can get on with her life — or not. One way or another, she wants to know. She is tired of waiting in limbo for the final verdict to come in. Like many of us, she had few or no symptoms when diagnosed, and was forced to transition abruptly from a life of wellness into the world of the sick. The endless journey continues as you desperately try to get back to normal, only to be treated as sick again during the follow up doctor visits. You're not only battling your own doubts and uncertainties, but you find yourself living in a world that doesn't come in agreement with your healing. You're anxious to move on with your life, but you find yourself struggling with the same doubts and questions as Carla.

There may be a new normal that sets in after a close encounter with death and the destruction it brings into your life. But there is also a new life that comes when you walk with Jesus through the rubble. This new life is better than the old. In the old life, you cowered in fear when the enemy threatened to take back what your God has won for His glory. You agreed with a world that treated you like you you're still sick and your future is uncertain. In the old life, you waited under dark clouds of doubt, never certain of God's goodness, never sure you were really healed, just waiting for the enemy to rise up and confirm your worst fear.

There is a better way to live. If you belong to Christ, you are a brand new person. The old life is gone and a new life has begun! Your old life didn't just change when you reached out to Him. You were completely re-created. The life your parents gave you will come to an end, but you were born again into a new life that never ends. The sinful nature that we are all born with, that selfish nature that ruled your old life, was washed away by the saving work of Jesus. He saved you, not because of anything you did, but because of his mercy. He gave you this new birth and new life through the power of the Holy Spirit. Because of His grace, He declared you righteous and you now have access to eternity and all its treasures (Titus 3:5-7).

So, what does this mean for you today? It means that you have triumphed over sin and the threat of death through the power of Jesus (Romans 5:17-18). Death no longer has any hold over you because Jesus conquered it once and for all (1 Corinthians 15:54-55). You no longer walk in fear, but you walk in power, love, and a sound mind (2 Timothy 1:7). Overwhelming victory is yours, despite the trials and hardships of life (Romans 8:37). No fear, no worry, not the powers of hell or death itself will ever stop Him from loving you (Romans 8:38-39). You will never be alone because it's virtually impossible for Him to abandon you (Hebrews 13:5).

It means that you are God's masterpiece, created anew in Christ Jesus, so you can do the good things he planned for you long ago (Ephesians 2:10). He didn't save you for your own benefit, but for His. In your new life, the Holy Spirit gently guides you to step into your destiny and use your passions and gifts to save and serve the lost and hurting (Ephesians 4:12). For His glory alone, you give back to Him the very life He gave to you (Romans 6:13).

It means that you are under no obligation to go back to the old way (Romans 8:12). By the power of the Holy Spirit, your new, loving nature can resist evil and stand firm against worldly desires, temptations, and lies that want to hijack your life and come back into power again. With each victory, your trust in Him grows stronger, and your knowledge of Him deepens. As the Spirit continues to work, you become more and more like Jesus (2 Corinthians 3:18). There is no more waiting. It's time to move on with your new life. It's so much better than the old.

Father, thank you for my "new normal," my new life in Christ! By the power of your Spirit, help me to walk everyday in victory and bring glory and honor to your name. Amen.

EPILOGUE

PEACE FOR EACH HOUR

Now may the Lord of peace himself give you his peace at all times and in every situation. The Lord be with you all. — 2 Thessalonians 3:16

Last week, I had my annual mammogram and breast exam with the same doctor who removed the cancer from my breast in September, 1999. I thought my appointment time was 11:20 a.m. I was almost downtown when I realized it was actually scheduled for 11:40 a.m. The traffic was surprisingly light. I would be at least a half hour early and there was always a wait. Thankfully, I had my smart phone and could use the wait time to catch up on emails.

When I pulled up in front of the Cancer Center, I had my first hint there would be something very different about this appointment. Oddly, there were no other cars waiting in line. A smiling valet parking attendant ran out and opened the door for me. When I walked into the building, the elevator door was open, empty, and waiting. I stepped off the elevator on the 4th floor and entered the clinic. Soft feminine colors and beautiful artwork surrounded me as I checked in at the desk. Again, no line and no waiting.

I had no more removed my coat and settled into a comfy chair for a long wait when a cheerful, neatly dressed elderly woman called my name. We exchanged pleasant conversation as she escorted me back to the changing room and offered me a cup of coffee. I undressed and put on the dignified robe they provided (no sterile hospital gowns at this breast clinic!). When I opened the door, she was standing there waiting with my coffee in a china cup and invited me to have a seat in another beautifully decorated waiting room.

I was barely seated, when the x-ray tech came to get me for my mammogram. Six films later, after some sweet apologies for the discomfort, I had just returned to the waiting room when the nurse called me back for my doctor appointment. As she led me down the hall, my doctor was literally waiting for me outside the door of the examining room. Now I ask you, how often does this happen? She examined me and told me the radiologist had already read the films and everything looked great. I was out the door before my actual appointment time. I never had time to look once at my phone or take a sip of coffee, and my car was even waiting for me at the valet stand, warm with the engine running.

Wow. I asked the nurse where all the people were and she said they would see 175 patients in the breast clinic that day. Where were they? I breezed through the appointment on the wings of God's grace as if I were the only patient in the world, attended to by ministering angels from Heaven. It would be wonderful if my life always clicked along so smoothly. Unfortunately, it doesn't. And when it doesn't — when worry, fear, stress or some unpleasant circumstance threatens to steal my peace — I'm learning to immediately say four words: I trust you Jesus.

Through these words, I am immediately acknowledging His sovereign control over my life, and relinquishing mine. I am expecting Him to take care of my problem because I belong to God, He created me, and He cares for and maintains His creation (Psalm 5:3; Psalm 104:27-28). I am cultivating an abiding faith, a faith based on the promise that if I remain in Him and His words remain in me, I can ask Him for anything and He will provide (John 15:7). But mostly, by responding in trust, I can keep my peace. If I don't worry about anything, but instead, pray about everything; if I tell God exactly what I need, and thank him for all he has done, then I will experience God's peace that surpasses anything the human mind can understand (Philippians 4:6-7).

God's peace is a priceless gift, bought and paid for by the blood of His Son. It's a peace the world simply cannot give (John 14:27). The world's peace is tied to circumstances. You are at peace when things go smoothly and upset when they don't. You receive God's peace by trusting Him, regardless of your circumstances. You will always have problems in this imperfect world, but He has overcome the world (John 16:33). In Him, you have 24/7 access to a peace of such magnitude you cannot begin to grasp its scope and power. The next time circumstances threaten to steal your peace, say "I trust you Jesus" and fully expect Him to take care of it. Tell Him what you need and thank Him for setting the answers in motion. Now, may the Lord of peace give you His peace at all times and in every situation. The Lord be with you always.

Father, thank you for the priceless gift of peace that surpasses all human understanding. Regardless of the circumstances I encounter today, tomorrow, or the rest of my days on earth, I trust you Jesus. In you, I can have perfect peace, all day and every day — peace for each hour of the journey. Amen.

About the Author

Mary J. Nelson is an author, speaker, and Associate Pastor of Prayer and Freedom Ministries at Hosanna! Church, a church of over 6500 members in Lakeville, MN. She has a passion for helping people encounter God and His goodness in the midst of trials and be empowered and set free to live out their destiny. She emerged from a breast cancer diagnosis in 1999 eager to share how God restored and transformed her life. Her deepest desire is to give away what she has freely received.

Mary is the author of *Grace for Each Hour: Through the Breast Cancer Journey* (Bethany House, 2005) and *Hope for Tough Times* (Revell, 2009). Her books inspire those suffering from cancer, broken relationships, unemployment, financial failure, or devastating loss by helping them draw close to the heart of God. She founded and leads the Pray for the Cure cancer healing and discipleship ministry at Hosanna! where she also serves as a leader in the Sozo inner healing ministry. She and her husband, Howie, have two adult children and two grandchildren, and have been married for 36 years. They enjoy exploring the country together on their Gold Wing motorcycle and are leaders in Hosanna! Bikers, a ministry that reaches over 600 fellow bikers.